SpringerBriefs in Modern Perspectives on Disability Research

Series Editors

Gabriel Bennett, Independent Researcher, Klemzig, Australia

Emma Goodall, Healthy Possibilities, Seaford, Australia

This book series on disability research is a comprehensive collection of research on disability and related issues. The series is designed to promote interdisciplinary collaboration and exchange, bringing together scholars and practitioners from different fields to share their perspectives and insights. Disability research is an interdisciplinary field that examines the social, cultural, historical, and political dimensions of disability. It encompasses a wide range of topics, including disability rights, accessibility, assistive technologies, healthcare, education, employment, and social welfare. Disability research scholars employ a range of theoretical and methodological approaches to understand the experiences of people with disabilities, as well as the ways in which disability intersects with other social identities such as race, gender, sexuality, and class.

The series seeks to advance knowledge and understanding of disability by publishing rigorous, innovative, and relevant research. It aims to promote disability rights and social justice by highlighting the ways in which people with disabilities are marginalized and discriminated against in society, and advocating for greater social inclusion and accessibility. The series also seeks to inform policy and practice by disseminating research findings that can help to shape policy decisions and contribute to positive social change.

Ramakrishnan Veerabathiran ·
Sheena Mariam Thomas

Disability Across Continents

Evolving Policies and Cultural Shifts in Asia and Africa

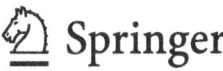

Ramakrishnan Veerabathiran
Human Cytogenetics and Genomics
Laboratory, Faculty of Allied Health
Sciences
Chettinad Hospital and Research Institute,
Chettinad Academy of Research
and Education
Kelambakkam, Tamil Nadu, India

Sheena Mariam Thomas
Human Cytogenetics and Genomics
Laboratory, Faculty of Allied Health
Sciences
Chettinad Hospital and Research Institute,
Chettinad Academy of Research
and Education
Kelambakkam, Tamil Nadu, India

ISSN 3004-9709 ISSN 3004-9717 (electronic)
SpringerBriefs in Modern Perspectives on Disability Research
ISBN 978-981-96-6075-9 ISBN 978-981-96-6076-6 (eBook)
https://doi.org/10.1007/978-981-96-6076-6

© The Editor(s) (if applicable) and The Author(s), under exclusive license to Springer Nature
Singapore Pte Ltd. 2025

This work is subject to copyright. All rights are solely and exclusively licensed by the Publisher, whether the whole or part of the material is concerned, specifically the rights of translation, reprinting, reuse of illustrations, recitation, broadcasting, reproduction on microfilms or in any other physical way, and transmission or information storage and retrieval, electronic adaptation, computer software, or by similar or dissimilar methodology now known or hereafter developed.
The use of general descriptive names, registered names, trademarks, service marks, etc. in this publication does not imply, even in the absence of a specific statement, that such names are exempt from the relevant protective laws and regulations and therefore free for general use.
The publisher, the authors and the editors are safe to assume that the advice and information in this book are believed to be true and accurate at the date of publication. Neither the publisher nor the authors or the editors give a warranty, expressed or implied, with respect to the material contained herein or for any errors or omissions that may have been made. The publisher remains neutral with regard to jurisdictional claims in published maps and institutional affiliations.

This Springer imprint is published by the registered company Springer Nature Singapore Pte Ltd.
The registered company address is: 152 Beach Road, #21-01/04 Gateway East, Singapore 189721, Singapore

If disposing of this product, please recycle the paper.

Preface

Disability is a multifaceted and universally relevant cultural, policy, economic, and technology issue. The experiences of people with disabilities (PwD) are profoundly shaped by the societal, cultural, and legislative frameworks of their regions, and this is particularly evident in the diverse and complex landscapes of Asia and Africa. These continents, characterized by their rich histories and cultural diversity, offer unique perspectives on how disability is perceived, addressed, and integrated within societies.

This book, "*Disability Across Continents: Evolving Policies and Cultural Shifts in Asia and Africa,*" explores the nuanced interplay of cultural beliefs, legislative progress, socioeconomic factors, and technological innovations in shaping the lived experiences of PwD. The book highlights the challenges and opportunities in fostering a more inclusive world by examining these factors through a comparative lens. The first section delves into the cultural dimensions of disability, tracing historical narratives, indigenous practices, and contemporary beliefs in Asian and African societies. These chapters shed light on how cultural contexts influence perceptions of disability and the ongoing shifts brought about by modernization and globalization. The second section focuses on the evolution of disability rights and policy. It examines the impact of global frameworks such as the UN Convention on the Rights of Persons with Disabilities (CRPD) while addressing national legislation, implementation challenges, and future pathways toward inclusivity. Socioeconomic challenges faced by PwD are addressed in the third section. This part emphasizes critical areas such as education, workforce participation, healthcare accessibility, and the enduring cycle of disability and poverty. By identifying systemic gaps and proposing actionable solutions, this section underscores the need for structural reforms. The fourth section focuses on technological innovations and their transformative potential for PwD in Asia and Africa. It explores advancements in assistive technologies, artificial intelligence, and telemedicine and the challenges of ensuring equitable access amidst a persistent digital divide. Finally, the book concludes with a focus on social inclusion and representation. From media portrayals to advocacy movements and from the unique challenges faced by PwD in conflict zones to building inclusive communities, this section emphasizes the role of societal attitudes and collective action in driving change. By weaving these interconnected themes, this book provides an in-depth understanding of the evolving dynamics affecting disability in Asia and Africa. It serves as a resource for scholars, policymakers, and advocates and a call to action to prioritize inclusivity and equality for all.

We intend for this book to provide valuable insights into the struggles and capabilities of individuals with disabilities in crises and the strategies used by humanitarian organizations to assist them.

Chennai, Tamil Nadu Ramakrishnan Veerabathiran
February 2025 Sheena Mariam Thomas

Acknowledgments The authors thank the Chettinad Academy of Research Education for their constant support and encouragement.

About This Book

Disability is a universal human experience intersecting with cultural, economic, and political structures across societies. Understanding how different regions perceive and respond to disability is crucial in fostering inclusive policies and practices. *Disability Across Continents: Evolving Policies and Cultural Shifts in Asia and Africa* offers a comprehensive exploration of the diverse challenges and opportunities faced by persons with disabilities (PwD) in these regions. By examining historical narratives, cultural attitudes, legal frameworks, socioeconomic factors, and technological advancements, this book provides valuable insights into the evolving landscape of disability rights and inclusion. Through a comparative lens, it highlights both the progress made and the persistent barriers, advocating for systemic change and collective action. This book serves as an essential resource for scholars, policymakers, and advocates committed to advancing disability rights and promoting a more equitable world.

Contents

1 **Cultural Perspectives on Disability in Asian and African Continents** 1
   1.1 Introduction 1
   1.2 Historical Treatment of Disability in Asian and African Continents 4
      1.2.1 Disability in Ancient Africa: Spiritual and Social Contexts 5
      1.2.2 Disability in Ancient Asia: Religious and Philosophical Interpretations 6
      1.2.3 Colonial Influences and the Shaping of Disability in Asia and Africa 8
      1.2.4 The Legacy of Historical Views on Disability 8
   1.3 Indigenous Knowledge and Traditional Practices 9
      1.3.1 Conventional African Perspectives Regarding Disability 10
      1.3.2 Traditional Asian Views on Disability 11
      1.3.3 The Function of Traditional Knowledge in Supporting People with Disabilities Today 13
   1.4 Current Cultural Views and Beliefs on Disability in Asia and Africa 13
      1.4.1 Disability in Asia: Cultural Views and Beliefs 14
      1.4.2 Disability in Africa: Cultural Views and Beliefs 14
      1.4.3 Contemporary Shifts and Advocacy in Both Regions 15
   1.5 Shifting Narratives: The Impact of Modernization 16
      1.5.1 Traditional Views vs. Modern Perspectives on Disability 16
      1.5.2 Globalization and the Influence of International Disability Rights Movements 17

		1.5.3	Technological Advancements and Accessibility Innovations	18

		1.5.3	Technological Advancements and Accessibility Innovations	18
		1.5.4	Economic Modernization and Employment Opportunities	19
		1.5.5	Education and Social Inclusion	19
		1.5.6	Cultural Shifts and the Rise of Disability Advocacy	20
	1.6	Conclusion		21
	References			21
2	**Disability Rights and Policy in Asian and African Continents**			27
	2.1	Introduction		27
	2.2	Evolution of Disability Rights: Global Influences and Local Adaptation		29
		2.2.1	1970s: Early Global Acknowledgment of Disability Rights	29
		2.2.2	1980: WHO Introduces ICIDH	29
		2.2.3	1981–1991: International Year and Decade of Disabled Persons	29
		2.2.4	1993: Adoption of the UN Standard Rules	30
		2.2.5	2001: Transition to the ICF Framework	30
		2.2.6	2006: Adoption of the CRPD	30
		2.2.7	Global Disability Rights Movement	30
		2.2.8	Evolution in Asia	31
		2.2.9	Evolution in Africa	31
	2.3	National Legislation: Progress and Remaining Gaps		32
		2.3.1	Disability Rights and Laws in the Asian Continent	33
		2.3.2	Disability Rights and Laws on the African Continent	38
	2.4	Policy Implementation Challenges and Solutions		41
	2.5	Conclusion		44
	References			44
3	**Socioeconomic Challenges Faced by People with Disabilities in Asia and Africa**			47
	3.1	Introduction		47
	3.2	Availability of Education and Standard of Services		49
	3.3	Workforce Inclusion and Economic Empowerment		54
	3.4	Healthcare and Rehabilitation: Gaps in Accessibility		57
	3.5	Breaking the Link Between Disability and Poverty		60
	3.6	Conclusion		65
	References			66

4	**Technological Innovations and Their Impact on Disability in Asian and African Continents**	69
	4.1 Introduction	69
	4.2 Assistive Technologies: Progress and Barriers	71
	4.3 AI and Robotics: Future of Accessibility	74
	4.4 The Role of Telemedicine and Digital Health	77
	4.5 Overcoming the Digital Divide: Equitable Access to Innovations	83
	4.6 Conclusion	85
	References	86
5	**Social Inclusion and Representation in Asian and African Continents**	91
	5.1 Introduction	92
	5.2 Disability in Media, Arts, and Sports	94
	5.3 Advocacy Movements and Leadership by Young Activists	98
	5.4 Disability in Conflict Zones and Humanitarian Crises	100
	5.5 Building an Inclusive Society: Pathways Forward	103
	5.6 Conclusion	107
	References	107
Appendices		111

Abbreviations

4IR	Fourth Industrial Revolution
ADLER	Activities of Daily Living Exercise Robot
ADLs	Activities of Daily Living
AGR	Augmented Reality
AI	Artificial Intelligence
AIDS	Acquired Immunodeficiency Syndrome
AR	Assistive Robotics
ASCEND	Asian Collaboration for Excellence in Non-Communicable Disease
AT	Assistive Technologies
BCIs	Brain-Computer Interfaces
CAGR	Compound Annual Growth Rate
CAR	Central African Republic
CBR	Community-Based Rehabilitation
CDPF	China Disabled Persons Federation
CEDAW	Convention on the Elimination of All Forms of Discrimination Against Women
CERD	Convention on the Elimination of All Forms of Racial Discrimination
COVID-19	Coronavirus Disease 2019
CPOA	Continental Plan of Action
CRPD	Convention on the Rights of Persons with Disabilities
DAL	Digital Academic Literacy
DPOs	Disabled People's Organizations
DPSA	Disabled People in South Africa
EFA	Education for All
e-health	Electronic Health
ERWs	Explosive Remnants of War
ESCAP	Economic and Social Commission for Asia and the Pacific
FUE	Federation of Uganda Employers

HICs	High-Income Countries
HIV	Human Immunodeficiency Virus
ICF	International Classification of Function
ICFD	International Classification of Functioning and Disability
ICIDH	International Classification of Impairments, Disabilities, and Handicaps
ICT	Information and Communication Technologies
ICU	Intensive Care Unit
IDD	Intellectual and Developmental Disabilities
IDPs	Internally Displaced Persons
IE	Inclusive Education
IL	Information Literacy
ILO	International Labour Organization
INDS	Integrated National Disability Strategy
ISCED	International Standard Classification of Education
IT	Information Technology
JONAPWD	Joint National Association of Persons with Disabilities
LMICS	Low- and Middle-Income Countries
LPPD	Law on Protection of Persons with Disabilities
MDGs	Millennium Development Goals
ML	Machine Learning
NCPEDP	National Centre for Promotion of Employment for Disabled People
NDHSA	National Digital Health Strategies and Frameworks
NGO	Non-Governmental Organization
NUDIPU	National Union of Disabled Persons of Uganda
OECD	Organisation for Economic Co-Operation and Development
PDA	Persons with Disabilities Act
PEPUDA	Promotion of Equality and Prevention of Unfair Discrimination Act
PRC	People's Republic of China
PWD	Person with Disability
QR	Quick Response
RCTs	Randomized Controlled Trials
RPWD	Rights of Persons with Disabilities
SDG	Sustainable Development Goals
SEN	Special Educational Needs
SSA	Sub-Saharan Africa
SSNs	Social Safety Nets
TB	Tuberculosis
TCM	Traditional Chinese Medicine
UN	United Nations
UHC	Universal Health Coverage
UNESCAP	United Nations Economic and Social Commission for Asia and the Pacific

UNHCR	United Nations High Commissioner for Refugees
UNICEF	United Nations Children's Fund
UWC	University of the Western Cape
VR	Virtual Reality
WHO	World Health Organization

List of Figures

Fig. 1.1 An infographic illustrating various types of disabilities. It is divided into four categories: Physical, Mental, Sensory, and Intellectual Disabilities. Physical Disabilities include amputation, arthritis, and spinal cord injury. Mental Disabilities feature bipolar disorder, Alzheimer's disease, and Parkinson's disease. Sensory Disabilities cover blindness, deafness, and loss of taste. Intellectual Disabilities include Down Syndrome, Prader-Willi syndrome, and brain injury. Each category is visually represented with corresponding images 2

Fig. 1.2 Different perceptions surrounding disability in Asia and Africa. On the left, under "Disability in Asia," it highlights spiritual interpretations like Hinduism, Buddhism, and Confucianism, family and community-based care in countries like India, China, and Japan, and conventional medical procedures such as Ayurveda and traditional Chinese medicine. On the right, under "Disability in Africa," it discusses spiritual significance as a curse or divine punishment, community support systems, and traditional healing practices involving spiritual ceremonies and shamans. A central figure symbolizes the shared human experience of disability 7

Fig. 2.1	Disability-related laws in selected African and Asian countries. The image is a map highlighting disability legislation in selected African and Asian countries. On the left, Africa includes Uganda with laws from 1995, 2003, and 2020; Kenya with laws from 2010, 2003, and 2006; and South Africa with laws from 1997, 1998, and 2000. On the right, Asia features China with laws from 1990 and 1994; India with laws from 1987, 1995, and 2016; and Bangladesh with laws from 1972, 2001, and 2013. The map visually separates the continents and lists key disability-related acts for each country	41
Fig. 3.1	Illustration of the global goals of sustainable development (This figure illustrates key Sustainable Development Goals (SDGs) to foster an inclusive and equitable society. The central theme, Reduced Inequalities, emphasizes the need for accessibility and equal opportunities for all, including persons with disabilities. These elements highlight the interconnected efforts required to promote a fair, sustainable, and inclusive world. The visual representation reinforces the importance of global collaboration in achieving these objectives)	55
Fig. 4.1	Map illustration of technological innovations in Asia and Africa. The figure illustrates the technological advancements in assistive technology for people with disabilities across Asia and Africa. The left side represents Asian innovations, including AI-powered wheelchairs, prosthetic hands, brain-computer interfaces, AI hearing aids, and prosthetic lenses. The right side highlights African assistive technologies, such as the ShazaCin App, the IXAM platform for visual impairments, AI-powered magnifiers, smart bracelets, and advanced prosthetic limbs. The central AI symbol signifies the role of artificial intelligence in enhancing accessibility and independence for individuals with disabilities in both regions	74

List of Figures

Fig. 5.1 Concept of social inclusion for individuals with disabilities (It highlights community participation, emphasizing integrating people with disabilities into society. Accessible transportation is depicted as a crucial factor in ensuring mobility through adapted vehicles. The role of AI in assistive technology is also showcased, demonstrating how AI-powered innovations enhance accessibility and independence. Additionally, the image includes wheelchair accessibility, underscoring the importance of inclusive infrastructure. It also acknowledges neurological and motor disabilities, representing the challenges faced by individuals with movement disorders. Furthermore, elderly and mobility support are depicted through assistive devices like walkers, catering to seniors and individuals with limited mobility) 93

List of Tables

Table 1.1	The cultural perspectives, modern beliefs, specific societal views, and actions taken regarding disability in Asia and Africa	17
Table 3.1	Key challenges and aspects of inclusive education for PwDs across different regions	62
Table 4.1	Various software developments designed to enhance accessibility for people with disabilities in public spaces	78
Table 5.1	Global disability rights issues, focusing on civic engagement, intersectionality, and policy advocacy	104

Chapter 1
Cultural Perspectives on Disability in Asian and African Continents

Abstract This chapter explores the complex cultural perceptions of disability in Asia and Africa, highlighting the interplay of historical, spiritual, and contemporary factors that shape societal attitudes and experiences. In these regions, disability has traditionally been viewed through a spiritual and cultural lens, often linked to ancestral beliefs, divine intervention, or karmic retribution, resulting in both reverence and marginalization of individuals with disabilities. As globalization, urbanization, and modernization have progressed, new frameworks for understanding disability have emerged, influenced by international human rights standards and advocacy. This shift toward more inclusive, human rights-based approaches is particularly evident in urban centers, though traditional communities may resist these changes due to deeply rooted cultural values. The chapter examines how these diverse cultural perspectives interact with modern concepts of disability, offering insights into the challenges faced by people with disabilities in rural and urban contexts. It underscores the importance of bridging the gap between tradition and progress to create inclusive societies that respect the rights and dignity of all individuals, regardless of ability.

Keywords Disability · Globalization · Advocacy · Social inclusion · And cultural diversity

1.1 Introduction

Despite being a common human experience, disability may be viewed, felt, and dealt with quite differently in different cultures and communities. The way that people with disabilities are viewed and incorporated into their communities is influenced by a complex web of cultural, historical, economic, and religious factors. These cultural perspectives on disability influence societal conventions, legislative frameworks, and even the experiences of individuals with disabilities all around the world. These viewpoints are vibrant, varied, and complex in Asia (Babik & Gardner, 2021) and Africa because they are shaped by spiritual worldviews, traditional beliefs, and the

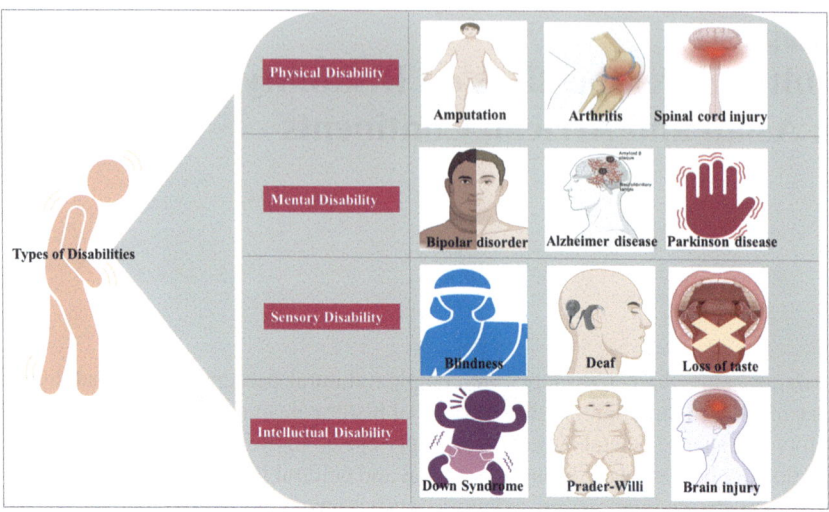

Fig. 1.1 An infographic illustrating various types of disabilities. It is divided into four categories: Physical, Mental, Sensory, and Intellectual Disabilities. Physical Disabilities include amputation, arthritis, and spinal cord injury. Mental Disabilities feature bipolar disorder, Alzheimer's disease, and Parkinson's disease. Sensory Disabilities cover blindness, deafness, and loss of taste. Intellectual Disabilities include Down Syndrome, Prader-Willi syndrome, and brain injury. Each category is visually represented with corresponding images

possibilities and problems associated with globalization and modernization (Barnes, 1985). The different types of disability are depicted in Fig. 1.1.

As is frequently the case in many Western situations, the cultural notion of disability in these two continents is not exclusively defined via a medical or individualistic perspective. Instead, more significant cultural, spiritual, and societal perspectives have frequently been used to understand and interpret disability. These viewpoints have a substantial influence on disability, influencing how people with disabilities negotiate their positions in society as well as how they are seen and treated. The lives of people with disabilities in Asia and Africa are influenced by deeply rooted customs and beliefs that have been handed down through the years. However, these perspectives are being challenged and reshaped by the quick changes brought about by modernization, urbanization, and global influences, creating a complicated conflict between tradition and development (Holzer et al., 1999).

Historical customs entwined with indigenous knowledge and religious beliefs form the basis of these cultural viewpoints. In both Asia and Africa, disability was frequently viewed through a supernatural or spiritual prism. Disability was considered in many communities as an indication of divine intervention, a manifestation of spiritual imbalance, or even the result of past-life activities. These ideas provided frameworks for comprehending disability and deciding how to treat those with impairments; they were not inherently destructive or immoral. Disability can be regarded as a sign of exceptional spiritual power or a rare gift, but it can also be perceived as a kind of divine retribution. People with disabilities had a special place in their societies because they were seen as a part of the more remarkable spiritual cosmic order, even though, in some cases, that role meant being marginalized (Ikechukwu & Asuquo, 2022).

This perception of infirmity as spiritually meaningful is especially noteworthy in many African civilizations, where ancestry, rituals, and community ties are essential to cultural activities. Disabilities, especially those affecting mental or cognitive capacities, were thought to be the consequence of ancestor spirits communicating through humans or by signs of spiritual importance in various African cultures. Because they were perceived as possessing spiritual insight or wisdom, people with disabilities were frequently revered due to this belief. In some cultures, disability was seen more pragmatically, with people and their families depending on support systems within the community. Disability was formerly viewed as a component of the diversity of human experience rather than something to be feared or scorned. However, there have also been instances where people with disabilities have faced prejudice because of their condition, have been marginalized, or have been excluded from social and economic activities (Okafor et al., 2022).

Similar to this, cultural and spiritual beliefs have long influenced how people in Asia see disabilities. The role of disability has been tightly linked to religious teachings like Buddhism, Hinduism, and traditional Chinese medicine in various regions of Asia, especially in China, India, and Southeast Asia. For instance, in Buddhism and Hinduism, the idea of karma frequently portrays disability as the outcome of deeds committed in past lifetimes. Individuals with disabilities may be viewed as having a unique spiritual function or purpose, or they may be perceived as suffering from the repercussions of previous transgressions. This knowledge affected how individuals with disabilities were treated as well as how they were included in their families and communities. With its focus on balancing mental, spiritual, and physical energy, traditional Chinese medicine also provided frameworks for treating disabilities, viewing them as imbalances in a person's overall health and physical limitations (Miles, 2013).

As these areas have developed, globalization and modernization have progressively influenced how people with disabilities view the world. Views on disability have changed in both Asia and Africa as a result of rapid urbanization, economic growth, and greater engagement with international human rights organizations. New frameworks for comprehending and resolving disability have emerged as a result of the increased awareness of disability as a social and human rights problem. One such framework is the CRPD, which advocates for more equality, accessibility, and inclusion for those with disabilities. In addition to helping to change cultural narratives, the growth of disability advocacy and awareness campaigns has also aided in dispelling long-held stigmas and misconceptions regarding disabilities. People with disabilities now have more options for social interaction, work, and education in metropolitan areas due to these improvements (Hiranandani & Sonpal, 2010; Munyi, 2012).

The modernization process is not without its complications, however. The communal, spiritually informed viewpoints that continue to predominate in rural and traditional communities clash with the trend toward more individualistic, medicalized understandings of disability in many Asian and African metropolitan centers. For instance, while policies of equality and inclusion for those with disabilities may be more prevalent in urbanized settings, rural communities may view these same policies as alien or incompatible with their cultural beliefs. Furthermore, people with disabilities and their families now face additional difficulties as a result of the quick economic development and growing expenses of social services and healthcare in these areas. The infrastructure and resources available to help people with disabilities may be scarce in many rural locations, where shifting economic realities may undermine conventional systems of care (Hiranandani & Sonpal, 2010). The experience of disability is being reinterpreted as these areas continue to negotiate the nexus of tradition and modernity. Disability is increasingly seen as a social phenomenon intricately linked to culture, identity, and human rights rather than just a medical condition. While modernization brings new possibilities for equality and inclusion, it also brings difficulties as long-standing cultural norms are challenged and reassessed. This has frequently resulted in more progressive policies and attitudes toward integrating individuals with disabilities into mainstream society and a more inclusive approach to disability in urban areas. However, in more conservative or rural regions, these shifts frequently clash with ingrained cultural values that still shape how people view disability (Bouin, 2018).

This chapter discusses how historical, spiritual, and contemporary factors combine to shape cultural perceptions of disability in Asia and Africa. Disability in these regions cannot be understood from a single perspective; instead, it is vital to recognize the diverse cultural, social, and economic contexts it encounters. By exploring the various cultural viewpoints on disability, this chapter aims to understand better the complex challenges that people with disabilities face in these areas. While traditional beliefs, modernization, and globalization still influence views toward disability, they are creating new opportunities for social engagement, equality, and inclusion. The ongoing challenge is to develop cultures that respect the rights and dignity of every person, regardless of ability, by bridging the gap between tradition and progress.

1.2 Historical Treatment of Disability in Asian and African Continents

The cultural, theological, and social structures that have molded Asia and Africa throughout the ages are intricately linked to how disability has historically been treated. With their diverse ethnic groups, dialects, and religious beliefs, both continents have distinctive perspectives on and approaches to disability. Some similar themes emerge, such as the significance of family and community, the effect of spirituality, and the junction of social hierarchy with disability, even though the lives of people with disabilities vary significantly among cultures and historical times.

1.2 Historical Treatment of Disability in Asian and African Continents

In Asia and Africa, disability was frequently seen as a complicated phenomenon connected to moral, social, and spiritual beliefs rather than just a physical problem. People's perceptions of disability were influenced by their spiritual interpretations, which included the idea that disability was a punishment from the gods, the outcome of ancestor wrath, or the result of karmic transgressions. Furthermore, whether they were marginalized or played unique roles of significance, people with disabilities were included in communal life in many ancient civilizations in ways that mirrored the larger ideals of society.

1.2.1 Disability in Ancient Africa: Spiritual and Social Contexts

Disability has traditionally been viewed through a spiritual or religious lens in many regions of Africa, with both positive and negative meanings. In traditional African communities, mental or physical disabilities were frequently associated with supernatural powers, ancestral spirits, or spiritual forces. In addition to being seen as a display of unique spiritual abilities, disability was also occasionally considered as a sign of divine disapproval or as a kind of retribution for ancestral transgression. As a result, people with impairments were frequently viewed as possessing a unique link to the supernatural or divine world, which inspired dread, awe, or admiration (Amadhila et al., 2024).

Disability was frequently associated with ideas of harmony and balance in the natural world in many African tribes. Traditional healers or spiritual leaders often aimed to restore this balance, since illness or incapacity was perceived as an imbalance in the spiritual or physical sphere. Through rituals, herbal medicines, or prayers, these healers would try to "cure" the patient by fusing their understanding of medicine with spiritual practices. A community's moral and spiritual strength may also be put to the test by disability, since how it responds to a disabled person is interpreted as a reflection of its ideals (Miles & Miles, 2018).

The treatment of people with disabilities was greatly influenced by the role that families and communities played. In many traditional African communities, care for people with disabilities was primarily the responsibility of the family, extended family networks, or even the larger village. Disability was not viewed as an isolated experience in these close-knit communities but as something that impacted everyone. To guarantee that people with disabilities were given their proper position in society, elders or other community leaders frequently played a crucial role. People with disabilities were commonly included in the community's social fabric, though to differing degrees, whether as revered participants in religious rites or as members who made non-monetary contributions to group activities (Bîrneanu et al., 2016; Bongo et al., 2018).

People with impairments were not always treated well by society, nevertheless. Disability was seen as a cause of shame and stigma in some civilizations, mainly when it came to severe physical or mental impairments. People with apparent disabilities were socially marginalized because they were occasionally viewed as a burden on the family or the community. Caste, class, or gender may also influence how people with disabilities are treated in a more hierarchical society. For example, because gender norms and expectations further complicate the perception of impairment, women with disabilities may have experienced more marginalization or lower status within the community (Gutterman, 2023).

1.2.2 Disability in Ancient Asia: Religious and Philosophical Interpretations

Many philosophical and theological traditions, including Buddhism, Taoism, Confucianism, and Hinduism, have had a significant impact on how people with disabilities are treated in Asia. For example, there are numerous references to disability in Hindu religious scriptures from ancient India, which are frequently interpreted through the prism of karma, the idea that people are born disabled as a result of their deeds in previous lifetimes. The Hindu religion holds that a person's current physical or mental disabilities are the consequence of sins or transgressions from past incarnations. Those born with impairments were frequently seen as getting what was considered just in this view, which saw disability as a moral and spiritual issue. However, this attitude did not always result in total social isolation (Avery, 2016; Wilson, 2019).

Furthermore, disability was entwined with ideas of purity and impure status in Hinduism, which has a strong legacy of caste and social duties. The lower castes, whose members were frequently viewed as worthy of their predicament because of previous transgressions or karma, may be connected to disability. However, infirmity has been viewed as a chance for spiritual development or metamorphosis in Hinduism. Despite their physical limitations, the disabled person may be able to achieve a higher level of spiritual awareness. It may result in respect in certain religious rituals or as a component of a spiritual path (Miles, 2013; Thapa et al., 2021).

Similarly, Buddhism offered a more complex perspective on disability as it expanded throughout Asia, reaching nations like China, Japan, and Southeast Asia. Buddhist philosophy believes that suffering is a natural aspect of existence and that everyone experiences a cycle of suffering, even those who are physically or mentally disabled. Buddhism, like Hinduism, holds that a person's previous deeds, or karma, determine their current situation in life, including their experience of handicap. Nonetheless, compassion and the reduction of suffering are highly valued in Buddhism. As a result, although there may not have been many institutional frameworks for care, Buddhist teachings frequently advocated for treating people with disabilities and urged society to view them with respect and compassion (McCormick, 2013).

1.2 Historical Treatment of Disability in Asian and African Continents

The concept of social harmony was essential to Confucianism's interpretation of handicap. Confucianism's emphasis on family values, societal obligations, and reverence for elders has resulted in a divided response to disability. Since they may be thought to be unable to carry out their social duties, people with disabilities may be viewed as a possible threat to societal cohesion. Confucianism, on the other hand, placed a strong emphasis on family responsibilities, and caring for disabled people was frequently seen as a moral requirement. Families were supposed to take care of disabled people, and in many situations, they were in charge of making sure that disabled people were acceptable (Qu, 2024).

Another significant philosophical movement in ancient China, Taoism, saw existence in terms of natural forces and equilibrium. It was common to understand disability as an imbalance or discord in the natural order. Some cultures encourage people with disabilities to seek balance and healing via natural means, including herbs, meditation, and physical activities. Taoist ideology also promoted the notion of living in harmony with nature. As a result, Taoism viewed disability as a spiritual ailment that could be treated by connecting with nature (Avery, 2016; Schumm & Stoltzfus, 2011). Figure 1.2 compares the perceptions, beliefs, and support systems surrounding disability in Asia and Africa.

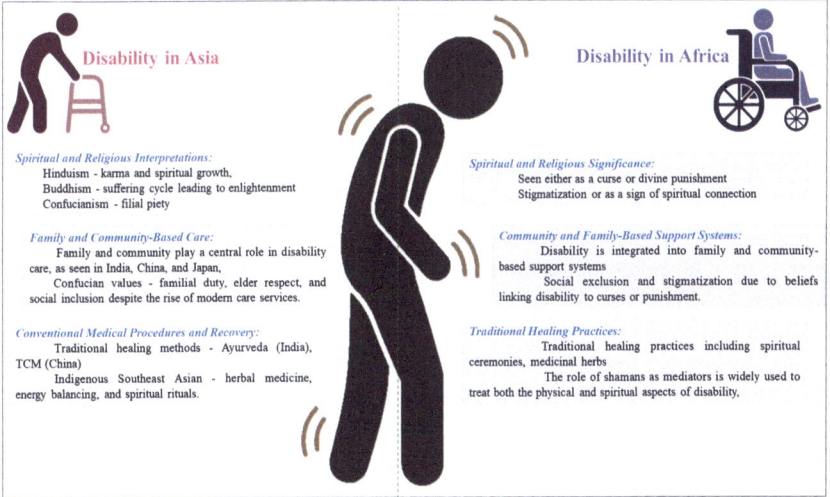

Fig. 1.2 Different perceptions surrounding disability in Asia and Africa. On the left, under "Disability in Asia," it highlights spiritual interpretations like Hinduism, Buddhism, and Confucianism, family and community-based care in countries like India, China, and Japan, and conventional medical procedures such as Ayurveda and traditional Chinese medicine. On the right, under "Disability in Africa," it discusses spiritual significance as a curse or divine punishment, community support systems, and traditional healing practices involving spiritual ceremonies and shamans. A central figure symbolizes the shared human experience of disability

1.2.3 Colonial Influences and the Shaping of Disability in Asia and Africa

The colonial era brought Western medical models and conceptions of disability that frequently conflicted with indigenous cultural understandings, which had a significant impact on how disability was historically treated throughout Asia and Africa. New establishments brought about by colonization, including schools, hospitals, and legal systems, started standardizing notions of disability following Western medical norms. This change signaled the start of a protracted process known as "medicalization," in which disability came to be seen as a disease that could be identified, managed, and frequently "cured" utilizing medical intervention (Ghosh & Bhaduri, 2024).

Western frameworks of disability, which prioritized individuality and medical classification, were frequently imposed in Africa by colonial forces. These frameworks clashed with indigenous peoples' more spiritual and community-centered conceptions of disability. Asylums and special schools were among the institutions created as a result of the colonial encounter that segregated people with impairments. These organizations, which were frequently impacted by the eugenics movements of the day, helped to create both physical and social hurdles to inclusion and strengthened the marginalization of people with disabilities (Ineese-Nash, 2020; Simbaya et al., 2019).

Although it manifested differently in each location, colonialism had a significant influence on disability in Asia as well. For instance, colonial policy in British India brought Western ideas of disability, which frequently ignored conventional medical systems like Siddha and Ayurvedic therapy (Buxton, 2018). The medicalization of disability, with a focus on "curing" (Hayes & Hannold, 2007) rather than adapting or integrating disabled people into society, was brought about by the establishment of Western-style hospitals and institutions. Similar care and educational methods that frequently separated people with disabilities from the larger society were enforced by colonial rulers in various regions of Asia (Konnoth, 2020).

The concept that disability was a flaw that needed to be corrected rather than a condition that could be adjusted or included in society was also brought about by Western colonization. The emphasis on individual therapy resulted in a reduction in traditional care methods that were based on community-based models, which had long-lasting repercussions on how persons with disabilities were treated socially in both Asia and Africa.

1.2.4 The Legacy of Historical Views on Disability

The way that impairments have historically been treated throughout Asia and Africa has had a lasting impact that still influences the lives of disabled persons in these places today. The way that disability is viewed and handled is still influenced by many indigenous beliefs and practices, even if colonization brought Western medical models and institutions. Disability is still frequently viewed via a complicated fusion of social, medical, and spiritual frameworks in Asia and Africa. Individuals with disabilities may face stigmatization, marginalization, or exclusion from both their communities and official institutions as a result of the conflicts between traditional and modern perspectives on disability (Foday & Sidikie, 2023).

Despite recent advancements, public attitudes and policies are still influenced by how disabilities have historically been treated in these areas. People with disabilities are still frequently seen as burdens in many regions of Asia and Africa, either because of the stigma that still surrounds infirmities or because of the difficulties brought on by insufficient infrastructure and services. However, there are growing attempts to incorporate people with disabilities into mainstream society as these areas rapidly modernize. These efforts include awareness campaigns, educational initiatives, and legislative reforms (Nagase, 1995).

A complex interplay of spiritual beliefs, social practices, and colonial legacies shapes the historical treatment of disability in Asia and Africa. While these regions have diverse approaches to disability, a common thread runs through the centuries of understanding disability as both a spiritual and social condition. As these societies continue to evolve, it is essential to acknowledge the historical context that has shaped contemporary attitudes and to work toward creating more inclusive environments that respect the dignity and rights of all individuals, regardless of ability.

1.3 Indigenous Knowledge and Traditional Practices

In Asia and Africa, the lives of people with disabilities have long been significantly shaped by indigenous knowledge and customs. Various knowledge systems have influenced how disability is perceived and dealt with on numerous continents because they are firmly anchored in regional cultures, religions, and social institutions. Indigenous knowledge systems often approach disability from a more holistic viewpoint, taking into account the physical, social, spiritual, and community components of an individual's well-being, in contrast to Western medical models of disability, which frequently concentrate on diagnosis, treatment, and rehabilitation. In addition to stressing the value of social integration and group support for people with disabilities, these traditional systems frequently underscore how intertwined people are with their families, communities, and the natural world (Eskay et al., 2012; Sande, 2022).

Disability is frequently viewed as a component of the larger social fabric rather than just a medical problem in Asia and Africa. Deeply ingrained cultural traditions and beliefs influence how people with disabilities integrate into their communities and their roles in families and society. In addition to providing care, these strategies aim to create opportunities for people with disabilities to contribute significantly to their communities' overall well-being. Therefore, in these areas, disability is frequently inextricably linked to more general ideas of social balance, human variety, and inclusion (Eskay et al., 2012; Miles, 2007).

1.3.1 Conventional African Perspectives Regarding Disability

Spiritual beliefs, community life, and the historical background of each ethnic group significantly impact traditional knowledge systems and practices around disability in Africa. Despite the tremendous cultural variation seen on the continent, specific general themes can be seen in how indigenous African communities view and deal with disability.

(a) Spiritual and Religious Significance: Many African societies use religious and spiritual frameworks to describe disability. Disability might be interpreted as a manifestation of spiritual energies, the outcome of ancestral misdeeds, or a message of divine disapproval. Some African groups, for instance, think that mental or physical infirmities are the consequence of a curse or retribution from the gods or spirits. People with impairments may be seen in these cultures as having been chosen by the spiritual world to bear the burdens of the spiritual world. Depending on how the community interprets it, this belief may lead to either veneration or stigmatization (Bondi, 2021).

However, not all traditional African communities have a bad opinion of people with disabilities. People with disabilities are viewed as possessing exceptional spiritual skills or endowments in some cultures. In some areas of West Africa, for example, people with impairments are believed to have a special bond with the spirit world and can communicate with ancestors or carry out jobs that others cannot. These people are occasionally held in high regard because of their alleged capacity to mediate between the material and spiritual worlds. Furthermore, some cultures view disabilities, particularly mental impairments, as indications of wisdom or as possessing unique skills that might advance the spiritual and cultural understanding of the group (Marini, 2011).

(b) Community and Family-Based Support Systems: Disability is frequently seen in indigenous African societies concerning family and community obligations. People with disabilities are usually cared for by community members and extended family members in these civilizations. This method emphasizes how African societies are collaborative, with the welfare of the society being entwined with that of the individual. As a result, disability is viewed as a problem that affects the entire family and community rather than as a singular experience (Puszka et al., 2022; Sam et al., 2023).

Their families and community roles greatly influence how people with disabilities experience life in providing care. Instead of being kept in institutions, people with disabilities are frequently incorporated into the community and given jobs or responsibilities that help the family or society as a whole operate. These responsibilities, which range among African civilizations, might involve participating in religious rites, carrying out significant cultural duties, or assisting in decision-making. According to several African civilizations, people with disabilities have unique tasks related to their condition, such as serving as spiritual and physical bridges or carrying out specific religious responsibilities (Hayes & Bulat, 2017).

Nevertheless, in many African communities, people with disabilities also experience social exclusion and stigmatization despite these community-based support networks. Families may attempt to conceal or isolate their disabled members in situations where disability is perceived as a curse or a punishment to escape the social stigma or shame attached to their condition. It might further marginalize disabled people by preventing them from accessing social, professional, and educational opportunities (Abberley, 1987; Trani et al., 2020).

(c) Traditional Healing Practices: In many African civilizations, traditional healing methods that include community engagement, spiritual ceremonies, and medicinal plants are used to alleviate disabilities. In the diagnosis and treatment of disability, traditional healers or shamans frequently play a key role. In addition to providing medical care, they mediate between the patient, their family, and the spiritual realm. Offerings to ancestors, prayers, or medicinal herbs are healing rituals that can treat infirmity's spiritual and physical reasons (Cumes, 2013).

Many people with disabilities in rural or indigenous areas still find great healing and support from these traditional therapies, even though they are frequently seen as a supplement to modern treatment. Particularly in places with inadequate healthcare infrastructure, traditional healing methods are often more readily available and less expensive than Western medical techniques (Berhe et al., 2024).

1.3.2 Traditional Asian Views on Disability

Spiritual beliefs, philosophical teachings, and communal institutions also influence indigenous knowledge and traditional behaviors related to disability throughout Asia. In Asia, like in Africa, disability is frequently viewed through the prism of holistic frameworks that take into account mental, spiritual, and physical health. Due to the impact of a vast range of cultures, religions, and philosophical traditions, these systems of thought differ significantly throughout the continent. Nonetheless, several recurring patterns show up, particularly concerning the impact of religious rituals and the function of community-based care (Babik & Gardner, 2021).

(a) Spiritual and Religious Interpretations: In many Asian cultures, spiritual and religious perspectives are frequently used to understand disability. Hinduism, for instance, often associates disability with the idea of karma, which holds that a person's current circumstances are shaped by their deeds in previous lifetimes. Therefore, it is frequently assumed that people with impairments are suffering as a result of their earlier crimes or transgressions. In contrast, infirmity is also seen as a chance for spiritual development or metamorphosis. It is possible to consider a person with a handicap on a spiritual path that enables them to develop qualities like compassion, humility, and patience (Schuelka, 2013).

Similar to this, disability is frequently viewed in Buddhism as a component of the cycle of suffering, which is a fundamental feature of the human condition. Buddhism holds that enlightenment may come from suffering, and people with impairments may be treated compassionately as they process their pain. In this sense, disability is something to be accepted as a component of the more significant process of spiritual development rather than something that has to be mended or cured. Since people with disabilities are fellow travelers on the path to enlightenment, Buddhist teachings exhort society to treat them with compassion and understanding (Bejoian, 2006).

The idea of filial piety, which highlights the value of family ties and reverence for elders, is frequently linked to the role of handicap in Confucianism. People with disabilities get considerate and respectful treatment, particularly from their relatives, who have a moral duty to see to it that their requirements are satisfied. Because social harmony and order are highly valued in Confucianism, people with disabilities may be assigned tasks that enable them to contribute to the family or community in ways that uphold this harmony (Canda, 2013).

(b) Family and Community-Based Care: Traditional Asian civilizations, like those in Africa, frequently strongly emphasize the family and community's role in treating disabilities. People with disabilities are expected to live with their families, where they will get assistance and be incorporated into the home, as the family is often viewed as the primary unit of care in many cultures. Collective responsibility for caring means that persons with disabilities are not isolated or alienated from everyday life in rural areas, where extended families commonly dwell together (Yan et al., 2014). For instance, family members often care for a disabled relative in India (Kalaiselvi et al., 2021). Extended families frequently reside in tight-knit communities where a person with a handicap does not always cause problems for the family or the community. The concept that a disability is a part of the social fabric of the family and community is reinforced by the community's support of the individual via social activities and everyday responsibilities (Yan et al., 2014).

The importance of the family is equally stressed in other Asian countries, including China and Japan. People with impairments, especially senior family members, are treated with respect and care because of the Confucian values of elder respect and familial duty. Despite the growing prevalence of contemporary care and social service institutions, these civilizations frequently feel the duty to care for disabled people within the family unit (Badanta et al., 2022).

(c) Conventional Medical Procedures and Recovery: In Asia, traditional healing methods also play a significant role in understanding and managing handicaps. For instance, Ayurvedic medicine, practiced for centuries in India, provides a comprehensive process for treating infirmities. Treating the entire person rather than simply the symptoms of a disability and balancing the body's energies are the foundations of Ayurvedic therapy. Therapies like yoga, massage, and herbal medicines are frequently utilized to treat the spiritual and physical components of disability (Mishra, 2003; Pandey et al., 2013).

Similarly, traditional Chinese medicine (TCM) in China uses the idea that qi, or vital energy, travels through the body to treat infirmity. TCM uses tai chi, herbal medicine, and acupuncture to try to balance the flow of qi. This energy flow is thought to be disrupted in people with disabilities, and traditional treatments are sought to bring the body back into harmony and balance. Southeast Asian conventional healing systems, including those in Thailand and Indonesia, combine herbal medication, physical therapy, and spiritual activities. In addition to employing herbs and other natural medicines to cure bodily ailments, traditional healers or shamans may undertake rituals to eliminate lousy energy or restore spiritual equilibrium in the individual (Jiang & Zou, 2013; Chaudhury & Rafei, 2002).

1.3.3 The Function of Traditional Knowledge in Supporting People with Disabilities Today

The treatment and care of people with disabilities still heavily relies on traditional knowledge and practices, even as contemporary Western approaches to disability have grown more common in both Asia and Africa. The primary source of assistance for disabled people and their families in many rural communities, where access to professional healthcare may be restricted, continues to be traditional wisdom.

Furthermore, conventional knowledge systems and contemporary methods frequently complement one another. Indigenous healing methods supplement official medical procedures in many Asian and African societies, resulting in a more comprehensive and integrated approach to disability care. A more complex view of disability that considers the condition's spiritual as well as physical aspects is made possible by this blending of traditional and modern approaches. The intricate interactions between spiritual, social, and medical understandings are reflected in the traditional practices and indigenous knowledge around disability throughout Asia and Africa. These customs, which have their roots in the spiritual and cultural beliefs of these areas, have influenced how people with disabilities are viewed and treated throughout history. Traditional knowledge systems continue to provide essential insights into how societies might develop more inclusive, supportive settings for people with disabilities despite the obstacles presented by industrialization and globalization.

1.4 Current Cultural Views and Beliefs on Disability in Asia and Africa

The way that disability is recognized and dealt with varies around the world according to cultural, historical, and social factors. Traditional views, religious ideology, socioeconomic standing, and access to healthcare and education all have an impact on how people see disability in various areas. With their vast cultural, linguistic, and traditional variety, Asia and Africa each provide unique perspectives on disability. There are significant variances across nations and areas within these continents, even while there are certain similarities in the way that disability is seen, particularly about social stigma and exclusion.

1.4.1 Disability in Asia: Cultural Views and Beliefs

Disability is still frequently viewed via a spiritual or religious prism in many Asian countries. For example, disability may be seen as a type of karmic retribution, divine punishment, or the result of ancestral misdeeds in nations like India (Kumari, 2019), Nepal (Hari, 2016), and Sri Lanka (Goyal, 2018). This idea may cause disabled people and their families to feel stigmatized and ashamed. On the other hand, some Buddhist and Hindu societies provide a more sympathetic viewpoint and see disability as a chance for spiritual development (Kayama et al., 2019). On the other hand, nations like China and South Korea, which Confucianism has heavily influenced, see disability in terms of societal peace and family prestige. Families may feel under pressure to conceal or minimize the existence of a disabled family member to avoid dishonor, as disabilities are frequently seen as sources of humiliation. Both the family and the individual may become socially isolated as a result (Canda, 2013).

The idea that disability is a medical disease that needs care, treatment, and rehabilitation is becoming more widely accepted in modern cultures and metropolitan areas. Disability is becoming more and more recognized in medical terms in nations like Malaysia, Singapore, and Japan with an emphasis on healthcare and rehabilitation as opposed to spiritual or supernatural origins. Stronger healthcare systems, laws, and societal initiatives encouraging the inclusion of people with disabilities all help this change (Disability, U.N., 2018).

Public perceptions are changing due to the growing activism for disability rights in Asia, primarily through international frameworks like the CRPD. The rights of disabled persons, including access to healthcare, work, and education, are increasingly being recognized in nations including Thailand, the Philippines, and India. Even while there is still a societal stigma, campaigning is progressively dispelling myths and promoting more accepting views of people with disabilities (Alwis, 2008).

1.4.2 Disability in Africa: Cultural Views and Beliefs

Disability is still frequently attributed to supernatural reasons in many African societies, such as witchcraft, divine retribution, or ancestors' wrath. According to conventional wisdom, disabilities might be brought on by evil spirits, which gives the impression that people with disabilities are cursed or that their families bear some responsibility. People with disabilities may be mistreated, socially isolated, and excluded as a result. Some cultures view disability as a sign of bad luck, and therefore, instead of seeking medical attention, families may turn to spiritual leaders or traditional healers for assistance. Some African communities, on the other hand, see disability as a sign of God's will or as a chance to show fortitude and resiliency. Because their diseases are seen as having spiritual importance, disabled people may be treated with some respect in these societies (Miles & Miles, 2018).

Both Islam and Christianity, which are extensively followed throughout Africa, often encourage empathy and consideration for those with impairments. With churches and mosques providing resources, support, and a sense of community for people with disabilities, many Christian and Muslim communities in Africa today promote inclusion. Since these religions place a strong emphasis on philanthropy and aiding the underprivileged, religious organizations frequently launch disability-focused programs to encourage the inclusion of disabled individuals (Unicef, 2012).

Even though disability rights are becoming more widely acknowledged, many African nations continue to believe that having a handicap is a sign of shame or bad luck. This is especially true in rural places, where traditional ideas are more ingrained. In these places, poverty and disability are frequently associated, and people may not be aware of the social or medical factors that contribute to impairment. People with disabilities may be further isolated from society by being excluded from family and community activities. Nonetheless, views are gradually shifting in metropolitan areas, mainly due to improved educational opportunities and the impact of international movements for disability rights. Organizations and activists attempt to counter negative preconceptions and encourage the inclusion of disabled persons in mainstream society (Campbell & Uren, 2011).

1.4.3 Contemporary Shifts and Advocacy in Both Regions

In both Asia and Africa, there is an increasing push for the rights and inclusion of people with disabilities. Advocacy groups, both local and international, have been instrumental in challenging outdated beliefs and pushing for policy reform. The ratification of the CRPD has been a significant factor in this shift, urging governments in both regions to adopt more inclusive laws and practices. Countries like Japan and South Korea have begun introducing disability-friendly policies in Asia, although there are still significant gaps, especially in rural regions. China has also made progress, but the deeply rooted cultural attitudes toward disability still create challenges. Similarly, in South Asia, India has made strides with the Rights of Persons with Disabilities Act, but social stigma and a lack of resources remain barriers. While progress has been slower in many parts of Africa, there has been a gradual shift in legal frameworks and public attitudes. South Africa's progressive disability rights laws serve as a model for other African nations.

Meanwhile, organizations such as the African Union are actively promoting the rights of people with disabilities, urging countries to ratify international conventions and integrate disability into national development policies. Despite these advances, people with disabilities in both regions continue to face challenges such as limited access to education, healthcare, and employment. The journey toward full inclusion is ongoing, but the growing influence of disability advocacy and the cultural and religious shifts toward greater compassion and understanding are beginning to reshape the landscape for people with disabilities in Asia and Africa. Table 1.1 outlines the cultural perspectives, modern beliefs, specific societal views, and actions taken regarding disability in Asia and Africa mainly highlighting the traditional and evolving perceptions and emphasizing the role of advocacy, legal reforms, and international influence in shaping inclusive policies and disability rights.

1.5 Shifting Narratives: The Impact of Modernization

Global society's modernization has resulted in significant shifts in every area, including how people with disabilities are perceived and treated. The effects of modernization on disability are becoming more and more noticeable in Asia and Africa, two continents with great cultural variety and complicated histories. These areas, which were formerly steeped in customs and beliefs around disability, are seeing a change in narratives due to globalization, technological development, worldwide campaigns for disability rights, and legislative changes. Because various nations in Asia and Africa are at different levels of development, this shift is not uniform. However, these continents' current view of disability has been formed by common patterns and difficulties (Miles, 2008).

1.5.1 Traditional Views vs. Modern Perspectives on Disability

Historically, superstition, religious interpretation, or a sense of social shame have been used to frame disability in many Asian and African societies. Disabilities were believed to be the outcome of one's past deeds, ill luck, or divine retribution in many old communities. Individuals with impairments were often excluded from society, kept out of the public eye, or even harmed. Disability, for instance, may have been connected to witchcraft, ancestral disapproval, or an unfavorable portent in rural African tribes, which may have led to traditional "cures" or seclusion. On the other hand, these perspectives are moving toward greater inclusion, human rights, and acknowledging disability as a social construct due to modernizing influences, especially those from the worldwide disability rights movement. The realization that disability is a mismatch between people and the social impediments they face rather than a fundamental weakness has contributed to this shift (Longchar & Cowans, 2014). Access, equality, and empowerment are becoming increasingly central to the discourse around disability as nations in Asia and Africa implement new laws, policies, and technological advancements.

1.5 Shifting Narratives: The Impact of Modernization

Table 1.1 The cultural perspectives, modern beliefs, specific societal views, and actions taken regarding disability in Asia and Africa

Region	Cultural views	Modern beliefs	Specific areas	Actions taken
Asia	In rural areas, disability is associated with bad luck or divine will	Increasing shift toward viewing disability through a medical lens (Japan, Singapore, Malaysia)	Traditional beliefs of disability as punishment for past deeds	Advocacy for inclusive policies through CRPD and local disability rights movements
	In Buddhist and Hindu societies, disability is viewed as a chance for spiritual growth	Emphasis on healthcare and rehabilitation, focusing on improving accessibility and inclusion	Confucian societies (China and South Korea) see disability as a source of family dishonor	Public awareness campaigns challenging traditional views, promoting disability rights
	In rural areas, disability is associated with bad luck or divine will	Globalization and international advocacy are shifting the view to human rights and inclusion	In some regions, disability is viewed as a stigma, leading to social isolation	Increasing legal protections for disabled individuals (e.g., rights to education and employment)
Africa	Disability is often attributed to witchcraft, divine retribution, or ancestral wrath	Shift toward viewing disability as a social construct, with emphasis on rights and empowerment	Poverty and disability are often linked, especially in rural communities	Advocacy groups countering stigma through education and legislative reforms
	Disability is seen as a curse, leading to mistreatment and exclusion in many communities	Influence of global disability rights movements, promoting equality and access to services	Disability is still associated with shame and bad luck in rural areas	Religious organizations advocating for empathy and inclusion for people with disabilities (e.g., Christian & Muslim efforts)
	Some cultures see disability as a sign of God's will or resilience, providing respect in certain cases	Increasing recognition of disability rights in urban areas due to international influences and modernization	In rural areas, traditional beliefs dominate views of disability	Local and international pressure for legal reform to ensure disabled people's rights (e.g., South Africa's disability laws)

1.5.2 Globalization and the Influence of International Disability Rights Movements

Modernization of disability narratives throughout the world has been dramatically influenced by the global disability rights movement, especially the 2006 adoption of the CRPD. Through the work of local advocacy groups and international organizations, fresh perspectives on inclusion, accessibility, and the rights of those with disabilities have been introduced to both Asia and Africa. For instance, the Philippines saw a significant legal change toward acknowledging the rights of people with disabilities in 1992 with the signing of the Magna Carta for Disabled Persons, which gave them more access to jobs, healthcare, and education. International lobbying activities and pressure from international organizations to bring national policies into compliance with the CRPD catalyzed this change. Laws like the Rights of Persons with Disabilities Act, 2016 have been adopted by several nations, including India, guaranteeing access to fundamental services and legal protection (Purcil, 2009).

Similarly, several African countries' ratification of the CRPD represented a dedication to enhancing the lives of those with disabilities. For example, discrimination based on disability is expressly forbidden under South Africa's constitution, and the nation has enacted several laws aimed at enhancing the lives of those with disabilities. These legal frameworks have changed the narrative from neglect and exclusion to empowerment and rights, even though implementing these laws has been sluggish in some areas (Fina, 2023).

1.5.3 Technological Advancements and Accessibility Innovations

It is indisputable that technology has shaped the lives of those with disabilities, especially in light of modernization. Technological developments have increased the opportunity for people with disabilities to participate in social life, work, and education in Asia and Africa. For many people with disabilities, assistive technologies like screen readers, mobility aids, and hearing aids have significantly enhanced their quality of life by enabling them to overcome some of the more conventional obstacles they had to overcome.

There has been a concentrated effort to integrate people with disabilities into society through innovative technology, accessible public transportation systems, and specialized educational resources in nations with highly developed technological innovation, such as South Korea and Japan. For instance, the government of South Korea has made significant investments in inclusive education systems and accessible technology, which has increased the number of individuals with disabilities in higher education and the workforce (Disability, U.N, 2018).

Due to differences in access to technology, the issue is more complicated in Africa. However, the widespread use of social media, mobile phones, and Internet access in cities has produced new venues for inclusion and campaigning. Previously unattainable educational resources, communities, and advocacy work are now accessible to those with impairments. For instance, many disabled persons in Kenya, both in urban and rural areas, have significantly benefited from using mobile technology for healthcare services, including healthcare information linked to impairments (Ehimuan et al., 2024).

1.5.4 Economic Modernization and Employment Opportunities

Productivity and labor involvement are given more importance due to economic modernization in Asia and Africa. The contribution that individuals with disabilities may provide to the workforce is increasingly acknowledged as both continents' economies continue to flourish. However, conventional perspectives continue to significantly affect public attitudes about disabilities in the workplace in many nations. People with disabilities have had fewer prospects for work and financial independence because of the perception that they are less able to contribute to the economy. Regarding integrating those with disabilities into the workforce, Japan has long been seen as a trailblazer in Asia. The scene has changed significantly due to laws mandating businesses to hire individuals with disabilities and government incentives for building accessible workplaces (Mwamadzingo & Chinguwo, 2015).

However, inclusive employment is still a problem in many African nations because of a lack of legal enforcement and widespread acceptance. Nonetheless, a few countries have achieved significant progress. For example, the Employment Equity Act of 1998 in South Africa requires equal opportunity for those with disabilities in the workplace, yet its implementation still has issues. Other African nations, including Nigeria and Kenya, have been gradually improving, especially in areas like information technology and education, where individuals with disabilities may carry out less physically taxing tasks and are more dependent on knowledge and skills (Das & Espinoza, 2019).

1.5.5 Education and Social Inclusion

Both Asian and African educational systems have been significantly impacted by modernization, with a growing focus on inclusive education. Children with impairments were frequently kept apart from regular classrooms in the past, either because of physical obstacles or because of societal perceptions that disability was an insurmountable obstacle. Regardless of ability, all children have the right to an education that satisfies their needs, according to the contemporary perspective on disability, highlighting the significance of inclusive education.

Asia has seen notable advancements in creating inclusive educational institutions in nations like Japan. For instance, to educate students with impairments, Japan has established a "special needs schools" system that collaborates with regular schools

(Cho & Park, 2024). The integration of children with disabilities into mainstream classes is encouraged by South Korean government policy, and teacher training programs have been extended to incorporate ways to meet a range of requirements (Kim, 2013).

But things are more complicated in Africa. The lack of facilities and qualified teachers is still a significant obstacle, even though certain nations, like South Africa, have made tremendous strides in integrating children with disabilities into regular classrooms. Children with disabilities sometimes have to rely on informal schooling or family care because special education programs are not readily available in many rural areas of Africa. However, the effects of modernization have also given rise to optimism, as new educational technology, international collaborations, and assistance from non-governmental organizations have opened up new avenues for inclusive education (Mpu & Adu, 2012).

1.5.6 Cultural Shifts and the Rise of Disability Advocacy

In addition to legal and technological developments, modernization has brought about cultural changes throughout Asia and Africa. A significant factor in the shift in perceptions of disability has been the emergence of grassroots and disability advocacy organizations. These movements have pushed for more inclusion and challenged antiquated ideas in the fight for the rights of individuals with disabilities domestically and globally (Pereira et al., 2016).

Through the planning of campaigns, training courses, and public awareness initiatives, advocacy organizations have dedicated their lives to promoting the rights of those with disabilities in both Asia and Africa. To guarantee that individuals with disabilities have access to public services, education, and employment, groups such as the National Centre for Promotion of Employment for Disabled People (NCPEDP) have been working in India (Shenoy, 2011). Organizations like the Disabled People's Act and the African Disability Forum have made significant progress in promoting inclusive legislation and increasing public awareness of the obstacles faced by those with disabilities in Africa.

The growth of social media and Internet platforms has also strengthened disability advocacy movements. People with disabilities use digital platforms to connect with others who have gone through similar things, share their stories, and raise awareness. The perception of disability has changed from charity to human rights and social inclusion, primarily due to this change in cultural narratives (Dube et al., 2006).

1.6 Conclusion

A complex interplay of historical, spiritual, and contemporary factors shapes the cultural perceptions of disability in Asia and Africa. These regions present a rich tapestry of beliefs and traditions that influence how disability is understood, experienced, and integrated into society. Traditional cultural and spiritual frameworks often position disability within a cosmic or ancestral context, leading to varying degrees of reverence, stigma, or exclusion. However, the rapid processes of globalization, urbanization, and modernization are challenging, and reshaping these long-standing views pushes toward more inclusive and human rights-centered approaches to disability. As these regions evolve, there is a growing recognition of disability as a social phenomenon intertwined with identity, culture, and human rights issues rather than just a medical or individual concern. The influence of global disability advocacy and the adoption of international frameworks such as the CRPD have spurred significant progress in urban centers, offering more excellent opportunities for equality, inclusion, and social participation for people with disabilities. Yet, in rural and more traditional communities, these changes often meet resistance as long-standing cultural values continue to shape attitudes and practices surrounding disability. The challenge lies in navigating the tensions between tradition and modernity, ensuring that new frameworks for understanding disability do not erase the importance of community, spirituality, and indigenous knowledge systems. Thus, it will be crucial to bridge these cultural divides, creating inclusive societies that honor the rights and dignity of all individuals, regardless of ability. By embracing the diversity of perspectives on disability, societies can foster environments where people with disabilities can thrive, contributing to a more equitable and just world for all.

References

Abberley, P. (1987). The concept of oppression and the development of a social theory of disability. *Disability, Handicap & Society, 2*(1), 5–19. https://doi.org/10.1080/02674648766780021

de Alwis, R. D. S. (2008). *Disability rights, gender, and development: A resource tool for action*. Wellesley Centers for Women.

Amadhila, E. M., John, H. C., Lawrence, L. J., & Rooy, G. V. (2024). Religion, culture, and disability in Namibia: Documenting lived experience of stigma and compulsory cure. *Journal of Disability & Religion, 28*(1), 57–86. https://doi.org/10.1080/23312521.2023.2255858

Avery, K. (2016). Disability and the three traditional Chinese belief systems: Buddhism, Taoism and confucianism.

Babik, I., & Gardner, E. S. (2021). Factors affecting the perception of disability: A developmental perspective. *Frontiers in Psychology, 12*, Article 702166. https://doi.org/10.3389/fpsyg.2021.702166

Badanta, B., González-Cano-Caballero, M., Suárez-Reina, P., Lucchetti, G., & de Diego-Cordero, R. (2022). How does confucianism influence health behaviors, health outcomes and medical decisions? A scoping review. *Journal of Religion and Health, 61*(4), 2679–2725. https://doi.org/10.1007/s10943-022-01506-8

Barnes, C. (1985). *Discrimination against disabled people (causes, meaning and consequences) or the sociology of disability* (Doctoral dissertation, Dissertation. https://www.pf7 d7vi404s1dxh27mla5569. https://www.wpengine.netdna-cdn.com/files/library/Barnes-Barnes-dissertation.pdf (22.03.2018).

Bejoian, L. M. (2006). Nondualistic paradigms in disability studies and Buddhism: Creating bridges for theoretical practice. *Disability Studies Quarterly, 26*(3). https://doi.org/10.18061/dsq.v26 i3.723

Berhe, K. T., Gesesew, H. A., & Ward, P. R. (2024). Traditional healing practices, factors influencing to access the practices and its complementary effect on mental health in sub-Saharan Africa: A systematic review. *British Medical Journal Open, 14*(9), Article e083004. https://doi.org/10.1136/bmjopen-2023-083004

Bîrneanu, A. G., Alexiu, T. M., Baciu, E. L., Sandvin, J. T., & Fylling, I. (2016). The role and influence of family and community relations on the disabled persons' labor market status: Perspectives of disabled individuals and family members. *Social Work Review/Revista de Asistenta Sociala, 15*(2).

Bondi, R. (2021). When disability strikes.

Bongo, P. P., Dziruni, G., & Muzenda-Mudavanhu, C. (2018). The effectiveness of community-based rehabilitation as a strategy for improving quality of life and disaster resilience for children with disability in rural Zimbabwe. *Jamba: Journal of Disaster Risk Studies, 10*(1), 1–10. https://doi.org/10.4102/jamba.v10i1.442

Buxton, H. (2018). *Disabled empire: race, rehabilitation, and the politics of healing non-white colonial soldiers, 1914–1940* (Doctoral dissertation, Rutgers University-School of Graduate Studies). https://doi.org/10.7282/T3B56P5Q

Campbell, A., & Uren, M. (2011). "The invisibles"... Disability in China in the 21st century. *International Journal of Special Education, 26*(1), 12–24.

Canda, E. R. (2013). Filial piety and care for elders: A contested confucian virtue reexamined. *Journal of Ethnic and Cultural Diversity in Social Work, 22*(3–4), 213–234. https://doi.org/10.1080/15313204.2013.843134

Cho, S., & Park, J. (2024). Inclusive education in Japan and its role in international cooperation: Analysis of a project for children with disabilities in Mongolia. *Asia Pacific Education Review, 25*(1), 229–242. https://doi.org/10.1007/s12564-023-09923-4

Cumes, D. (2013). South African indigenous healing: How it works. *Explore, 9*(1), 58–65. https://doi.org/10.1016/j.explore.2012.11.007

Das, M. B., & Espinoza, S. A. (2019). *Inclusion matters in Africa*. World Bank Group.

Della Fina, V. (2023). *The committee on the rights of persons with disabilities: Law and practice*. Springer Nature.

Disability, U. N. (2018). *Development report realizing the sustainable development goals by, for and with persons with disabilities.*

Dube, T., Hurst, R., Light, R., & Malinga, J. (2006). Promoting inclusion? Disabled people, legislation and public policy. *In and out of the mainstream.*

Ehimuan, B., Anyanwu, A., Olorunsogo, T., Akindote, O. J., Abrahams, T. O., & Reis, O. (2024). Digital inclusion initiatives: Bridging the connectivity gap in Africa and the USA–A review. *International Journal of Science and Research Archive, 11*(1), 488–501. https://doi.org/10.30574/ijsra.2024.11.1.0061

Eskay, M., Onu, V. C., Igbo, J. N., Obiyo, N., & Ugwuanyi, L. (2012). Disability within the African culture. *Contemporary voices from the margin: African educators on African and American education, 197–211.*

Foday, I., Sidikie, A. (2023). Influence of socio-cultural barriers on people with disability. https://doi.org/10.13140/RG.2.2.34288.23042

Ghosh, N., & Bhaduri, S. (2024). Creating disability as a category: Perspectives from West Bengal India. *Review of Disability Studies: An International Journal, 19*(3–4).

Goyal, N. (2018). *Disability in South Asia: Knowledge and experience* (A. Ghai, ed.).

Gutterman, A. S. (2023). *Disability and development*. Available at SSRN 4504319.

References

Hari, K. C. (2016). Disability discourse in South Asia and global disability governance. *Canadian Journal of Disability Studies, 5*(4), 25–62. https://doi.org/10.15353/cjds.v5i4.314

Hayes, A. M., & Bulat, J. (2017). *Disabilities Inclusive Education Systems and Policies Guide for Low-and Middle-Income Countries.* https://doi.org/10.3768/rtipress.2017.op.0043.1707

Hayes, J., & Hannold, E. L. M. (2007). The road to empowerment: A historical perspective on the medicalization of disability. *Journal of Health and Human Services Administration, 30*(3), 352–377. https://doi.org/10.1177/107937390703000303

Hiranandani, V., & Sonpal, D. (2010). Disability, economic globalization and privatization: A case study of India. *Disability Studies Quarterly, 30*(3/4). https://doi.org/10.18061/dsq.v30i3/4.1272

Holzer, B., Vreede, A., & Weigt, G. (1999). *Disability in different cultures: Reflections on local concepts* (p. 384). Transcript Verlag. https://doi.org/10.14361/9783839400401

Ikechukwu, K., Asuquo, G. *Dialogue on African religion, culture and development: Proceedings of the 2022 international conference of the association for the promotion of African studies.* https://doi.org/10.13140/RG.2.2.15475.81447

Ineese-Nash, N. (2020). Disability as a colonial construct: The missing discourse of culture in conceptualizations of disabled Indigenous children. *Canadian Journal of Disability Studies, 9*(3), 28–51. https://doi.org/10.15353/cjds.v9i3.645

International panel on social progress, & Bouin, O. (2018). Rethinking society for the 21st century: Report of the international panel on social progress. *Cambridge University Press.* https://doi.org/10.1017/9781108399661

Jiang, Y., & Zou, J. (2013). Analysis of the TCM theory of traditional Chinese health exercise. *Journal of Sport and Health Science, 2*(4), 204–208. https://doi.org/10.1016/j.jshs.2013.03.008

Kalaiselvi, R., Parimala, L., & Manimegalai, B. (2021). Writing therapy on anxiety among differently abled adolescents. *International Journal of Creative Research Thoughts, 9*(2), 2320–2882.

Karalay, G. (2024). *Sociology of ageing: A South Asia perspective* (1st ed.). Routledge. https://doi.org/10.4324/9781003450214

Kayama, M., Johnstone, C., & Limaye, S. (2019). Adjusting the "self" in social interaction: Disability and stigmatization in India. *Children and Youth Services Review, 96*, 463–474. https://doi.org/10.1016/j.childyouth.2018.11.047

Kim, Y. W. (2013). Inclusive education in Korea: Policy, practice, and challenges. *Journal of Policy and Practice in Intellectual Disabilities, 10*(2), 79–81. https://doi.org/10.1111/jppi.12034

Konnoth, C. (2020). Medicalization and the new civil rights. *Ethics, Medicine and Public Health, 12*, Article 100435. https://doi.org/10.1016/j.jemep.2019.100435

Kumari, N. (2019). Karmic philosophy and the model of disability in ancient India. *Shanlax International Journal of Arts Science and Humanities, 7*(1), 39–43. https://doi.org/10.34293/sijash.v7i1.531

Longchar, A. W., & Cowans, G. (Eds.). (2014). *Doing theology from disability perspective.* Association for Theological Education in South East Asia (ATESEA).

Marini, I. (2011). The history of treatment toward persons with disabilities. In I. Marini, NM Glover-Graf, & J. Millington, J (Eds.), *Psychosocial aspects of disability: Insider perspectives and counseling strategies* (pp. 3–31). https://doi.org/10.1891/9780826180636

McCormick, A. J. (2013). Buddhist ethics and end-of-life care decisions. *Journal of Social Work in End-of-Life & Palliative Care, 9*(2–3), 209–225. https://doi.org/10.1080/15524256.2013.794060

Miles, M., & Miles, C. (2018). Disability in Africa: Religious ethical & healing responses, to and by people with disabilities, deafness, or mental debility: A bibliography through four millennia, with introduction and partial annotation.

Miles, M. (2007). Disability and deafness, in the context of religion, spirituality, belief and morality, in Middle Eastern, South Asian and East Asian histories and cultures: Annotated bibliography. Internet publication URLs: http://www.independentliving.org/docs7/miles200707.html and http://www.independentliving.org/docs7/miles200707.pdf.

Miles, M. (2008). Glimpses of disability in the literature and cultures of East Asia. *South Asia, the Middle East & Africa. A modern and historical bibliography.*

Miles, M. (2013). Buddhism and responses to disability, mental disorders and deafness in Asia-A bibliography of historical and modern texts with introduction and partial annotation, and some echoes in western countries. *West Midlands: UK.*

Mishra, L. C. (Ed.). (2003). *Scientific basis for Ayurvedic therapies.* CRC Press.

Mpu, Y., & Adu, E. O. (2021). The challenges of inclusive education and its implementation in schools: The South African perspective. *Perspectives in Education, 39*(2), 225–238. https://doi.org/10.38140/pie.v39i2.4583

Munyi, C. W. (2012). Past and present perceptions towards disability: A historical perspective. *Disability studies quarterly, 32*(2). https://doi.org/10.18061/dsq.v32i2.3197

Mwamadzingo, M., & Chinguwo, P. (2015). *Productivity improvement and the role of trade unions. A Workers' Education Manual.*

Nagase, O. (1995). *Difference, equality and disabled people: Disability rights and disability culture.*

Okafor, I. P., Oyewale, D. V., Ohazurike, C., & Ogunyemi, A. O. (2022). Role of traditional beliefs in the knowledge and perceptions of mental health and illness amongst rural-dwelling women in western Nigeria. *African Journal of Primary Health Care & Family Medicine, 14*(1), 1–8. https://doi.org/10.4102/phcfm.v14i1.3547

Pandey, M. M., Rastogi, S., & Rawat, A. K. S. (2013). Indian traditional ayurvedic system of medicine and nutritional supplementation. *Evidence-Based Complementary and Alternative Medicine, 2013*(1), Article 376327. https://doi.org/10.1155/2013/376327

Pereira, E., Kyriazopoulou, M., & Weber, H. (2016). Inclusive vocational education and training (VET)–Policy and practice. In *Implementing inclusive education: Issues in bridging the policy-practice gap* (pp. 89–107). Emerald Group Publishing Limited. https://doi.org/10.1108/S1479-363620168

Purcil, L. (2009). *Monitoring the human rights of persons with disabilities: laws, policies and programs in the Philippines.* Disability Rights Promotion International.

Puszka, S., Walsh, C., Markham, F., Barney, J., Yap, M., & Dreise, T. (2022). Community-based social care models for indigenous people with disability: A scoping review of scholarly and policy literature. *Health & Social Care in the Community, 30*(6), e3716–e3732. https://doi.org/10.1111/hsc.14040

Qu, X. (2024). Confucianism and human rights-exploring the philosophical base for inclusive education for children with disabilities in China. *Disability & Society, 39*(6), 1443–1464. https://doi.org/10.1080/09687599.2022.2143324

Roy Chaudhury, R., & Muchtar Rafei, U. (2002). *Traditional medicine in Asia.*

Sam, R. K., Pillay, S., & Ngcamu, B. S. (2023). The role of family and community support system in improving the lives of people with disabilities in South Africa. *Journal of Public Administration, 58*(4), 1142–1153. https://doi.org/10.53973/jopa.2023.58.4.a17

Sande, N. (2022). *African churches ministering "to and with" persons with disabilities: Perspectives from Zimbabwe.* Routledge. https://doi.org/10.4324/9781003256335

Schuelka, M. J. (2013). A faith in humanness: Disability, religion and development. *Disability & Society, 28*(4), 500–513. https://doi.org/10.1080/09687599.2012.717880

Schumm, D., & Stoltzfus, M. (2011). Beyond models: Some tentative Daoist contributions to disability studies. In *Disability and Religious Diversity: Cross-Cultural and Interreligious Perspectives* (pp. 103–122). Palgrave Macmillan US. https://doi.org/10.18061/dsq.v30i3/4.1284

Shenoy, M. (2011). Persons with disability and the India labour market: Challenges and opportunities. *ILO, 13*(1).

Simbaya, J., Shakespeare, T., Nyariki, E., & Mugeere, A. (2019). Success in Africa: People with disabilities share their stories. *African Journal of Disability, 8*(1), 1–7. https://doi.org/10.4102/ajod.v8i0.522

Thapa, R., Van Teijlingen, E., Regmi, P. R., & Heaslip, V. (2021). Caste exclusion and health discrimination in South Asia: A systematic review. *Asia Pacific Journal of Public Health, 33*(8), 828–838. https://doi.org/10.1177/10105395211014648

References

Trani, J. F., Moodley, J., Anand, P., Graham, L., & Maw, M. T. T. (2020). Stigma of persons with disabilities in South Africa: Uncovering pathways from discrimination to depression and low self-esteem. *Social Science & Medicine, 265*, Article 113449. https://doi.org/10.1016/j.socscimed.2020.113449

Unicef. (2012). Partnering with religious communities for children.

Wilson, A. (2019). Barriers and enablers provided by Hindu beliefs and practices for people with disabilities in India. *Christian Journal for Global Health, 6*(2), 12–25. https://doi.org/10.15566/cjgh.v6i2.250

Yan, K. K., Accordino, M. P., Boutin, D. L., & Wilson, K. B. (2014). Disability and the Asian culture. *Journal of Applied Rehabilitation Counseling, 45*(2), 4–8. https://doi.org/10.1891/0047-2220.45.2.4

Chapter 2
Disability Rights and Policy in Asian and African Continents

Abstract This chapter scrutinizes the complex coaction of disability rights and policy in Asian and African nations. It analyzes the historical development of international disability rights frameworks, highlighting their influence on national legislation. The study contrasts the progress made in several legal frameworks in Asian and African countries with the significant challenges remaining in implementation. These challenges include persistent societal stigma, inaccessible infrastructure, limited access to education and employment, and resource constraints. The paper emphasizes the importance of community-based rehabilitation (CBR), inclusive education, and accessible transportation in achieving meaningful inclusion for persons with disabilities (PwDs). Finally, it underscores the requisite for bespoke solutions that deliberate these regions' inimitable cultural, socioeconomic, and infrastructural contexts to actualize disability rights and create fully inclusive societies.

Keywords Disability · Rights · Policies · Rehabilitation · And communities

2.1 Introduction

The fundamental principles of the personal liberties mission are grandeur, sovereignty, equality, and solidarity, which are essential in the context of disability and the broader pursuit of justice and inclusion (Bruce et al., 2002). These principles provide the foundation for protecting individuals from the misuse of power and fostering the growth of the human spirit. However, in inaccessible or ableist societies, the foundational rights of PwDs are frequently infringed upon, necessitating more excellent protection and recognition of their rights (Fernandez et al., 2017).

PwDs, widely acknowledged as the most prominent global minority group, face significant challenges, including low educational attainment, limited job opportunities, high rates of poverty, and poor health. They are disproportionately subjected to abuse and violence and frequently lack knowledge about their rights and available resources (Harpur, 2012). Even with progress in disability advocacy and protective laws by the close of the twentieth century, the monetary and diplomatic status of PwDs continues to be vulnerable, especially in the global South (Meekosha & Soldatic, 2011).

In high-resource nations, social safety nets (SSNs) and rehabilitation programs are typically well-established, providing crucial support for individuals with disabilities. However, in middle- and low-resource nations, these services are often absent, leaving individuals with disabilities to struggle with everyday tasks without government-sponsored aid (Hartley & Tarvydas, 2022). The situation is further exacerbated by societal attitudes that frequently portray disabilities as intrinsically harmful, framing people with disabilities as mere recipients of charity and disregarding their rights (Harpur, 2012).

Globally, the prevalence of disability has risen alongside increasing life expectancy. According to the 2011 WHO World Disability Report, Africa exhibits a higher prevalence of severe and moderate disabilities among younger demographic groups (under 60 years old) compared to many other regions, driven by factors such as infectious diseases and injuries, despite limited literature on the subject (Cannata et al., 2022).

Asia, with its vast population of nearly 4 billion people, accounts for approximately 60% of the 650 million people with disabilities worldwide (Thongkuay, 2009). Asian nations, characterized by their diverse socioeconomic and cultural contexts, face unique challenges and opportunities in addressing disability and mental health issues (Akram et al., 2024). Cultural factors in some Asian societies contribute to the stigmatization of disability, with disabilities often attributed to past-life transgressions. Such stigmas may extend to the entire family, creating additional barriers to inclusion and empowerment (Parker, 2001).

Urban accessibility further illustrates the challenges faced by PwDs. Inaccessible urban infrastructure perpetuates social exclusion, diminishes the standard of existence, and relegates PwDs to "incomplete citizenship." The degree of inclusion in urban environments is influenced by social and physical factors, government structures, disability rights initiatives, and cultural and economic settings (Chou et al., 2024).

In numerous low- and middle-income countries (LMICs), social protection plays an ever-growing role in poverty alleviation efforts, primarily through non-conducive abet programs like cash transfers and in-kind benefits. The importance of social security is highlighted by its inclusion as a specific target under the Sustainable Development Goals (SDGs) Poverty Goal, which aims to ensure broad coverage for the poor and vulnerable and establish nationally suitable social protection systems and measures for everyone, including basic safety nets, by 2030. However, despite growing global attention on disability inclusion in development, relatively little is known about integrating people with disabilities into social protection systems. It includes both disability-specific programs (focused primarily on people with disabilities) and mainstream social protection programs (targeted at the general population or specific groups but not explicitly at people with disabilities) (Walsham et al., 2019). Addressing these challenges underscores the pressing need for disability rights and

2.2 Evolution of Disability Rights: Global Influences and Local Adaptation

policies that ensure equity and inclusion, particularly in the Asian and African continents, where unique cultural, socioeconomic, and infrastructural contexts demand tailored solutions.

The history of disability rights has evolved through significant milestones in international frameworks, social movements, and regional adaptations. This section provides a chronological narrative to explore these developments, particularly in Asia and Africa.

2.2.1 1970s: Early Global Acknowledgment of Disability Rights

The 1970s represented a pivotal moment in establishing disability rights internationally. During this time, the UN adopted the Declaration on the Rights of Mentally Retarded Persons and the Declaration on the Rights of Disabled Persons, setting forth principles that recognized the rights of PwDs. However, these credentials primarily mirrored a medical and charitable perspective, which reinforced paternalistic attitudes that were subsequently contested by the disability community (Gostin, 2000).

2.2.2 1980: WHO Introduces ICIDH

In 1980, the WHO launched the International Classification of Impairments, Disabilities, and Handicaps (ICIDH), which categorized impairments, disabilities, and handicaps. Despite criticisms for its individualistic perspective, the ICIDH standardized health surveys globally, paving the way for more nuanced frameworks (Mayhew, 2003).

2.2.3 1981–1991: International Year and Decade of Disabled Persons

1981, the UN proclaimed the International Year of Disabled Persons, followed by the International Decade of Disabled Persons from 1982 to 1991. These initiatives raised global awareness about disability-related issues and urged governments to implement the World Programme of Action Concerning Disabled Persons in 1982. This program focused on rehabilitation, prevention, and ensuring equivalent prospects for PwDs (Patterson, 2024).

2.2.4 1993: Adoption of the UN Standard Rules

In 1993, the UN General Assembly approved the Standard policies ensuring the Equalization of Opportunities for PwDs. Those rules provided a discretionary framework to guide policy development and international cooperation. They highlighted the roles of the states in ensuring equality and promoting global partnerships to advance disability rights (Lang, 2009; Stein &Lord, 2021).

2.2.5 2001: Transition to the ICF Framework

In 2001, the WHO superseded the ICIDH with the International Classification of Functioning, Disability, and Health (ICF). The ICF incorporated social and ambient conditions into its analysis of disability, marking a shift toward a holistic understanding of the interaction between health and society (Mayhew, 2003).

2.2.6 2006: Adoption of the CRPD

The UN Convention on the Rights of Persons with Disabilities (CRPD) was implemented in 2006, marking a significant milestone in history. Acknowledging disability as a human rights dispute, the CRPD integrated societal development and human rights principles to promote inclusion and independence for PwDs. This framework catalyzed a reorientation in global and regional approaches to disability rights (Rioux, 2011).

2.2.7 Global Disability Rights Movement

Since the 1970s, people with disabilities have driven the Universal Disability Rights Movement, challenged traditional views, and advocated for inclusion. This movement emphasized the social construal of disability, highlighting environmental and communal barriers rather than individual impairments as the main obstacles to participation (Hughes, 2009; Sabatello & Schulz, 2014).

2.2.8 Evolution in Asia

In Asia, regional efforts have aligned with global frameworks to advance disability rights.

2.2.8.1 Asia-Pacific Decades of Persons with Disabilities (1993–2012)

The Asia-Pacific Decade of PwDs (1993–2002) initiated regional collaboration to eliminate barriers to participation and equality. This was succeeded by the second Decade (2003–2012), emphasizing legal reforms and establishing oversight institutions (UNESCAP).

2.2.8.2 Biwako Millennium Framework for Action (2002) and Biwako Plus Five (2007)

These frameworks called for removing discriminatory laws, ensuring impartiality, and enhancing the participation of individuals with disabilities. They emphasized institutional support and policy implementation for sustainable progress.

2.2.8.3 Adoption of the CRPD and Optional Protocol (2006)

By 2010, several Asian nations, including Azerbaijan, Bangladesh, China, India, and Thailand, had ratified the CRPD. Countries like Mongolia and Nepal joined the Optional Protocol, allowing individuals to address rights violations through UN mechanisms. However, the absence of a regional human rights court in Asia has hindered enforcement efforts, compounded by debates over "Asian values" and global human rights principles.

2.2.9 Evolution in Africa

2.2.9.1 Contributions to the CRPD Development

African delegations, including those from Sierra Leone, Comoros, Mali, Uganda, Morocco, South Africa, and Cameroon, significantly contributed to the foundational text of the CRPD. Experts from Algeria, Kenya, and Tunisia played vital roles in shaping the treaty, reflecting Africa's commitment to global disability rights frameworks (Onazi, 2024).

2.2.9.2 Ratification of the CRPD and Optional Protocol

Currently, 46 African countries have consented to the CRPD, and 33 have also endorsed the Optional Protocol, which allows individuals to submit complaints directly to the UN Committee on the Rights of PwDs. These commitments illustrate the region's substantial alignment with international standards (Nigussie Koski, 2021).

2.2.9.3 The African Decade for PwDs (1999–2019)

The African Union declared 1999–2009 as the African Decade for PwDs, later extended to 2010–2019. The Continental Plan of Action (CPOA), espoused in 2013, mirrored CRPD provisions while addressing Africa-specific contexts. The African Commission also expanded its mandate in 2009 to include disability rights alongside those of older persons (Lord et al., 2013).

2.2.9.4 Challenges and Resource Constraints

Despite aligning with the CRPD, the African Decade for Persons with Disabilities faced significant resource constraints, resulting in unmet objectives. This underscores the need for strategies tailored to Africa's unique challenges and regional disparities (African Union Commission, 2015).

2.3 National Legislation: Progress and Remaining Gaps

National disability policies are a determining factor in recognizing the experiences and societal contributions of PwDs by protecting their individual and collective rights (Fernandez et al., 2017). While general human rights frameworks include sustenance for PwDs, disability-specific policies are essential. Historically, these frameworks provided only minimal protection, as the construal of traditional human rights instruments often failed to account for the unique rights of PwDs (Leshota, 2013). This underscores the pressing need for enhanced recognition and safeguards, especially in societies shaped by inaccessibility and ableism. The rise of the disability justice movement and the growing recognition of the communal example of disability have brought disability policy to the forefront of policy discussions. In addition to securing fundamental human rights, disability policies highlight the meaningful contributions of PwDs to cultural, communal, and fiscal spheres (Harpur, 2012). Their implementation signals a government's obligation to advance the rights of PwDs while fostering collective efforts toward social progress that is both measurable and inclusive (Vaughn, 2003).

2.3 National Legislation: Progress and Remaining Gaps

National governments issue public policies as a means of directing attention toward particular areas (like housing, education, employment, and health), problems (like climate change, the COVID-19 response, and peace and security), or segments of the populace (like women and girls, indigenous people, older people, and people with disabilities). Public policies can be used for several purposes, such as setting guidelines, outlawing specific behaviors, controlling sectors or behaviors, allocating or redistributing resources, encouraging innovation and other acts, and influencing public perception of a given topic or problem (UNESCAP, 2022).

2.3.1 *Disability Rights and Laws in the Asian Continent*

2.3.1.1 India

All lawful citizens of India are equally covered by the Indian Constitution, regardless of their physical or mental disabilities. The constitution guarantees the following fundamental rights to PwDs:

- The constitution guarantees all individuals, including PwDs, the right to equal status and opportunity, liberty of thought, belief, expression, faith, worship, and the advancement of human dignity.
- The government is prohibited from discriminating against any Indian citizen, including those with disabilities, based on race, religion, social status, sex, or place of birth by Article 15(1).
- According to Article 15(2), no members, including those with disabilities, shall be subject to any of the aforementioned limitations, constraints, or circumstances concerning their use of bathing ghats, wells, roads, tanks, or public resorts that are maintained entirely or in part with public funds or for the general public's use, or concerning their entry to dining spots, inns, stores, and public amusement venues.
- No one can be treated as an untouchable, even those with disabilities, regardless of their status. Article 17 of the Constitution states it would be a crime with legal penalties.
- Article 21 of the Constitution ensures the safeguarding of personal existence and freedom for all individuals, including those differently-abled individuals.
- Article 45 of the Constitution mandates that each child, including those with impairments, is guaranteed free and compulsory education from the State until they reach the age of 14. No child can be denied admission to any state-run school or financial aid based on race, caste, religion, or language.
- The Hindu Succession Act of 1956, about Hindus, states that a person's physical deformity or impairment does not preclude them from inheriting their ancestors' property.

- Similarly, no clause prevents people with disabilities from inheriting an ancestral asset under the Indian Succession Act of 1925, which governs testamentary and intestate succession.

In addendum to the above, PwDs are guaranteed equality, dignity, and access to opportunities in several other rights of life by the Indian Constitution (Bhattacharyya, 2014).

(a) *The Mental Health Act, 1987*

The following rights are granted to mentally ill people by the Mental Health Act of 1987:

(i) *Rights of patients with mental illness*: Including the rights of individuals with mental health issues in the preamble of the Mental Health Act (1987) helps address the violation of rights experienced by mental health patients. The family, not the government, is the primary caregiver in India; hence, these rights should be balanced with the family's rights. It's also important to consider the stress on caregivers and the lack of resources for mental illness in India. Even juveniles and inmates with mental illnesses are entitled to care in government-run psychiatric institutions or nursing homes.
(ii) *Right to health*: For those who suffer from mental illnesses, this entails having access to high-quality mental health services as well as adequate physical and mental health treatment. Only by implementing the National Mental Health Program can this be possible. Thus, the emphasis must change from "respect," "promote," and "protect" to "fulfill" (Math et al., 2011).

(b) *The Persons with Disabilities Act, 1995*

To put into action the "Proclamation on the Full Participation and Equality of the People with Disabilities in the Asian and Pacific Region," the PwD (Equal Opportunities, Protection of Rights, and Full Participation) Act was enacted in 1995. Visual impairment, low eyesight, locomotor disability, auditory impairment, mental retardation, mental illness, and leprosy recovery were the seven conditions of disability included in the Act. The Act had a social fortune tactic for PwD, primarily focusing on early disability detection and prevention, PwD education, and PwD employment. The Act also made a 3% reservation in government positions and educational institutions possible. As a non-discrimination measure, it strongly emphasizes creating barrier-free environments (Narayan & John, 2017).

(c) *The Rights of Persons with Disabilities Act, 2016*

Cerebral palsy, muscular dystrophy, dwarfism, hard of hearing, acid attack victims, speech and language disabilities, autism spectrum disorders, specific learning disabilities, chronic neurological disorders like multiple sclerosis (Balakrishnan et al., 2019) and Parkinson's disease (Jagadeesan et al., 2017), blood disorders like thalassemia, sickle cell anemia, and hemophilia, and multiple disabilities are now included in the list, which was increased from seven to twenty-one conditions by the RPwD

Act of 2016. "A condition marked by considerable limitations in intellectual abilities (such as reasoning, acquisition of knowledge, and problem-solving) and adaptive behavior, which encompasses a variety of everyday relational and practical life skills, including certain intellectual disabilities and autism spectrum disorders," is the definition of intellectual disability, which replaces mental retardation as the nomenclature. A person is considered to have a benchmark disability if they have at least 40% of the above disabilities. PwDs validated under section 58(2) of the Act need high support. The RPwD Act of 2016 states, "The relevant Government shall assure that PwDs enjoy the same rights as others, including equality, a life of dignity, and respect for their integrity." Additionally, section 3 specifies that no PwD should face discrimination based on disability unless it is proven that the Act or omission in question is a reasonable means of accomplishing a legitimate objective. No individual can be imprisoned solely because of their disability. The government is responsible for ensuring that Pwds can live in the community and must act to provide reasonable accommodations (Balakrishnan et al., 2019).

2.3.1.2 China

The medical paradigm of impairment is still widely accepted in China, as seen by the conceptual and semantic shifts around disability. Article 2 of Order No. 36 (1990) of the President, which established the Law of the PRC on the Protection of PwDs of 1990, provided the formal definition of a disabled person. Since 1995, China's Disability Identification Card, issued based on the unchanged China Practical Disability Determination Standard, has been the primary means of identifying persons with disabilities (classified into seven categories) for resource allocation. While still in effect, this standard determines disability based on listed impairments and is used in most relevant laws and policies (Hao & Li, 2020).

China's Law on the Protection of Disabled Persons, first espoused in 1990 and amended in 2008, establishes a national framework for disability policy. The law covers six key areas: education, rehabilitation, cultural life, employment, social security, and accessibility. These areas define data collection on disability, structure provincial regulations, and inform annual reports and action plans. While the organizational structure remains consistent between 1990 and 2008, the amended law reflects a more compassionate and generous approach to state support for disabled persons.

- The State Council Executive Order establishes the legislative guidelines for developing a nationwide system for the prevention and rehabilitation of disabilities. The document outlines the twin duties' first job as being integrated into China's current social service infrastructure, specifically the National Economic and Social Development Plan, the fundamental public service system, and policies aimed at reducing poverty (Article 4).

- Community rehabilitation clinics will serve as the hub of a national rehabilitation service system that will offer rehabilitation counseling, daily living skills training, rehabilitation nursing care, and assistive equipment fitting (Article 20).
- The "Disabled Persons' Education Regulations" mandate that governments at all levels of government, as well as businesses and social groups, hire disabled people to increase work possibilities (Articles 2–4).
- It mandates all employing units to have a goal of hiring disabled people to make up at least 1.5% of their total workforce, in addition to making broad appeals (Article 8).
- The hiring percentage is 25% of the total workforce for special employment units with a large concentration of disabled people (Article 11).
- The rules also forbid employers from discriminating against disabled people in hiring, advancement, academic rank determination, compensation, social security, and living welfare (Article 13). Employers must also give disabled people job transition, orientation, and reorientation training (Article 14).
- Additionally, these employing units, particularly those that serve disabled people, will be given preference when the government purchases their goods and services (Article 18).

China ratified the UNCRPD in 2008, and its national policy for PwDs is integrated into the 13th Five-Year Plan (2016–2020). The Constitution guarantees equality and the freedom to work for all citizens, ensuring that persons with disabilities receive State and societal support, including social insurance, medical services, and material assistance. The Law on Protection of Persons with Disabilities (LPPD) (1990) is the primary statute safeguarding civil rights, promoting equality in education, employment, and welfare, and prohibiting discrimination in recruitment, employment, promotion, and other areas (UNESCAP, 2023).

2.3.1.3 Bangladesh

Bangladesh faces enormous challenges in defending its rights since PwDs embrace a sizable section of the population. In Bangladesh, an estimated 16 million people, or 10% of the total population, have a disability. Every nation's citizen is guaranteed fundamental human rights under the Constitution of the People's Republic of Bangladesh, regardless of ethnicity, gender, religion, or other characteristics. It also forbids discrimination of any kind against people with disabilities or other social groups (Islam & Jahan, 2018). Bangladesh's high disability incidence is said to be caused by several divisors, including overcrowding, severe poverty, illiteracy, ignorance, and, most importantly, a dearth of access to healthcare and services. PwDs have difficulty participating in social events, work, school, and every facet of life. In the social, cultural, and occupational spheres, disabled people can participate equally with the proper state resources. Thus, the government of Bangladesh has implemented disability laws and taken disability rights problems seriously (Islam & Juhara, 2021).

2.3 National Legislation: Progress and Remaining Gaps

(a) ***The Constitution of the People's Republic of Bangladesh (1972)***

Every citizen, including those with impairments, must be treated equally under the country's constitution. PwDs are guaranteed the right to work and education under the Bangladeshi constitution. Article 15 of the Bangladeshi Constitution highlights the importance of education and other basic essentials. A unified, universal, and widely applicable educational system is the goal of Article 17, which emphasizes the commitment to free and compulsory education. By connecting education with social requirements and producing citizens who are sufficiently trained and motivated to solve those needs, it aims to give all children a free, vital education. It also highlights the need to eradicate illiteracy within a legally mandated deadline. According to Article 28, no citizen may be excluded from public areas, recreational facilities, or educational establishments based on religion, caste, race, gender, or any other condition, limitation, or disability. While Article 29 forbids bias based on sex, caste, religion, race, or place of birth in public service or employment, Article 27 guarantees everyone's right to equal treatment under the law. Additionally, Article 31 provides the fundamental right to legal protection and fair treatment for all citizens and individuals in Bangladesh. Any conduct that endangers a person's life, liberty, body, reputation, or property is declared illegal (Neety, 2023).

(b) ***Bangladesh Persons with Disability Welfare Act, 2001***

To safeguard the rights and dignity of PwDs and encourage their involvement in national and social contexts, the Bangladesh Persons with Disability Welfare Act, 2001, was established.

The Act emphasizes:

- Developing evidence-based data on disabilities.
- Promoting preventive measures and providing affordable care services for PwDs through healthcare facilities.
- Ensuring access to inclusive education.
- Promoting skill development and vocational training for PwDs.
- Establishing an inclusive and supportive work environment.
- Providing adequate nutrition for PwDs.
- Introducing credit-support programs to aid in rehabilitation.
- Facilitating accessible transportation and movement infrastructure.

The Act highlights the necessity of mass media efforts to foster an inclusive and supportive atmosphere for PwDs. It also covers measures for PwDs' food support, access to sufficient medical supplies, and healthcare services. However, some contend that rather than empowering PwDs in community-based settings, this emphasis on nutrition and healthcare promotes an institutionalized approach to care. The Act also includes financial assistance, which aims to create rehabilitation facilities and pay for rehabilitation expenses. Along with vocational training, it advocates for attempts to match PwDs with appropriate jobs based on their skills. Additionally, reserved quotas for PwDs in the workforce are legally mandated, especially in government employment. Notably, the administration lacked accurate data on the number of PwDs in the nation when the law was tabled in Parliament. Detractors have questioned how a comprehensive program could be formed without correct data, and this lack of trustworthy statistics has been a primary source of controversy. Furthermore, rather than taking a rights-based approach that emphasizes inclusion and empowerment, the Act has come under fire for mainly depending on the medical and charitable conceptions of disability (Haque, 2020).

(c) *The Rights and Protection of Persons with Disability Act of 2013*

In line with the United Nations Convention on the Rights of Persons with Disabilities (UNCRPD), the Bangladeshi government passed the Rights and Protection of Persons with Disabilities Act on October 9, 2013. This Act replaced the previous Disability Welfare Act of 2001, marking a shift from a welfare-based model to a rights-based approach to address the needs and concerns of PwDs. The passage of this law was driven by extensive advocacy efforts from human rights advocates, civil society organizations, and Disabled Peoples' Organizations (DPOs), whose persistent efforts played a pivotal role in enacting this progressive legislation. The Act offers hope for bettering the lives of PwDs in Bangladesh. It establishes their rights and provides a framework for efficient defense and advancement. Establishing several committees at the regional and national levels is a crucial aspect of the Act. By guaranteeing improved legal implementation and protecting PwDs' rights, these committees hope to promote a more just and inclusive society (Nuri et al., 2022).

2.3.2 Disability Rights and Laws on the African Continent

2.3.2.1 South Africa

(a) *Integrated National Disability Strategy (INDS)*

In November 1997, South Africa adopted the White Paper on an Integrated National Disability Strategy (INDS), grounded in the social model of disability. This signaled a change from welfare and medical models, which see disabled people as dependent and unproductive, to a framework that encourages equality and inclusion. The INDS provides guidelines for nondiscriminatory development planning, program execution, and service delivery. Although the INDS is not yet law, government agencies must include its provisions in their disability policies and programs. The national and provincial governments are implementing their suggestions. South Africa has also passed laws that address the rights of PwDs. These include mainstream laws that benefit disabled people and specific rules on social security, education, employment, and training (Dube, 2005).

(b) *Employment Equity Act*

Discrimination against PwDs is a common theme in the literature and is frequently caused by unfavorable attitudes and ignorance. Prejudicial attitudes can result in discriminatory behavior, and one of the main obstacles to lowering this kind of discrimination in PwD employment is a lack of knowledge. PwDs are often viewed as inferior by those without disabilities, which feeds into workplace discrimination, leading to unemployment and poor working conditions (Maja et al., 2011). The Employment Equity Act aims to improve employment prospects for historically underrepresented groups by addressing workplace discrimination against them. It recognizes the differences in income, occupation, and employment brought about by apartheid and other forms of discrimination. The Act gives people the right to pursue justice if they have been the victims of unfair discrimination, directly or indirectly. Race, gender, handicap, sexual orientation, religion, HIV status, and other factors are among the grounds for discrimination. The Act aims to end discrimination brought on by any employment policy or practice by advancing equal opportunity (Thabethe, 2022).

As stated in the preamble, the Employment Equity Act seeks to:

- Encourage true democracy and defend the equality guaranteed by the Constitution.
- Get rid of unfair workplace discrimination.
- Put in place workplace equity policies to mitigate the effects of prior discrimination.
- Create a workforce that is varied and represents the general populace.
- Increase labor productivity and economic growth.
- As an International Labor Organization member, fulfill the Republic's obligations (Thabethe, 2022).

(c) ***Promotion of Equality and Prevention of Unfair Discrimination Act 2000***

Within the framework of the constitution, the Promotion of Equality and Prevention of Unfair Discrimination Act 2000 is a significant piece of legislation for PwDs. This Act is essential for recognizing how discrimination appears in society and, more significantly, for putting in place workable strategies to fight prejudice and promote equality (Dube, 2005).

First and foremost, the Promotion of Equality and Prevention of Unfair Discrimination Act (PEPUDA) satisfies the constitutional mandate to prevent and prohibit unfair discrimination. Second, it follows South Africa's international obligations, specifically those outlined in the International Convention on the Elimination of All Forms of Racial Discrimination (CERD) and the Convention on the Elimination of All Forms of Discrimination Against Women (CEDAW). Third, although significant progress has been made in equality jurisprudence since adopting the 1993 interim Constitution, discrimination continues to be a daily reality for many South Africans. Access to legal remedies has remained limited, primarily due to civil litigation's high costs and complexities. The new Act addresses this gap by offering accessible remedies, making justice more attainable for ordinary citizens rather than limited to the privileged few. Finally, the Act emphasizes equality as a fundamental pillar of South Africa's liberation ethos, comparable to the significance of liberty in the American constitutional framework (Pityana, 2003).

2.3.2.2 Kenya

An analysis of the laws governing access to justice for PwDs in Kenya outlines the innumerable sustenance of the legal framework, including the UNCRPD, the Constitution of Kenya 2010, and the Persons with Disabilities Act (PDA). These laws collectively address the rights of PwDs, ensuring their access to justice and equality within the legal system (Onyango, 2012).

(a) ***The Constitution of Kenya 2010***

The 1963 Kenyan Constitution lacked explicit protections against disability discrimination. This gap was bridged by the UNCRPD, domesticated in Kenya through the 2010 Constitution, which significantly advanced the rights of PwD. The 2010 Constitution guarantees dignity, equality, and fundamental freedoms for PwD, emphasizing social justice and mandating state interventions to support their full potential. Article 22 allows anyone to petition the courts on behalf of PwD for rights violations. Article 27 prohibits discrimination and ensures equality, while Article 28 upholds the inherent right to dignity for all, including PwD.

Key protections include fair administrative action, access to justice, and expeditious dispute resolution (Articles 48 and 50). Courts are required to address language barriers, offering interpreters when necessary. Article 54 specifically addresses PwD rights, ensuring dignity, accessible basic education, public spaces, transport, and information. It also guarantees access to Braille, sign language, and assistive devices, reinforcing inclusivity and equal participation (Wachira, 2021).

(b) ***UNCRPD***

Kenya is responsible for respecting and enforcing the UNCRPD's provisions as a party. The UN General Assembly implemented the UNCRPD on December 13, 2006, and Kenya ratified it in 2008. Notably, the drafting and passage of the PDA occurred while the UNCRPD was still being developed, with the PDA being enacted in 2003. One could argue that the enactment of the PDA marked a significant milestone for PwDs (Onyango, 2012).

(c) ***Persons with Disabilities Act 2003***

Kenya's first disability-specific law, the Persons with Disabilities Act (PDA) of 2003, forbids discrimination against PwDs and guarantees equal opportunity. It creates pertinent organizations, encourages inclusion, and lays a legislative framework to safeguard PwD rights. In addition, a 2019 amendment prioritizes environmental and societal constraints over individual potential. The National Council for PwD is established under Section 3 and is charged with registering PwD and related institutions, recommending policies, advocating for PwD rights, and liaising with government authorities. The Council manages welfare programs, enables housing and medical services, and guarantees accurate census statistics. It also offers advice on curriculum creation and infrastructural modifications to accommodate PwD.

According to the Act, PwDs can vote, participate in sports, work, and healthcare, and be educated in barrier-free surroundings. Section 11 requires the government to

2.4 Policy Implementation Challenges and Solutions

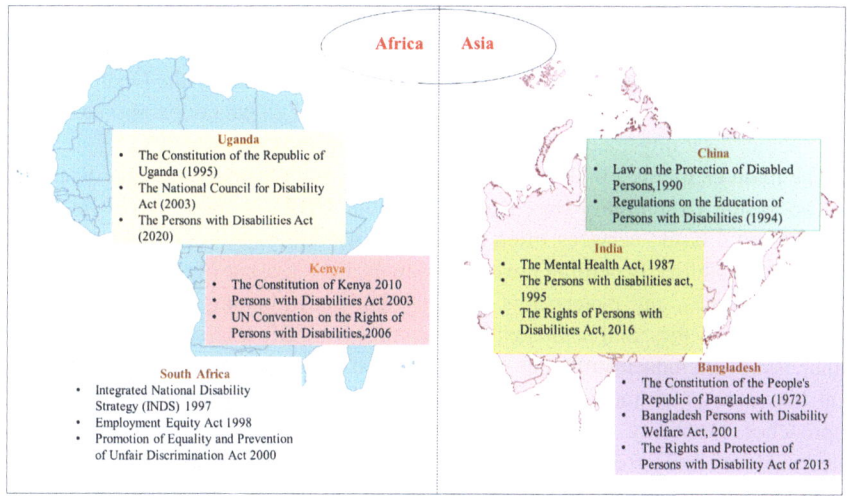

Fig. 2.1 Disability-related laws in selected African and Asian countries. The image is a map highlighting disability legislation in selected African and Asian countries. On the left, Africa includes Uganda with laws from 1995, 2003, and 2020; Kenya with laws from 2010, 2003, and 2006; and South Africa with laws from 1997, 1998, and 2000. On the right, Asia features China with laws from 1990 and 1994; India with laws from 1987, 1995, and 2016; and Bangladesh with laws from 1972, 2001, and 2013. The map visually separates the continents and lists key disability-related acts for each country

allocate resources for these rights to be fully realized. PwD legal representation in court proceedings is covered under Section 38, which requires pro bono services, fee waivers, and accessible court facilities. The Chief Justice controls the rules governing interpreters and the prompt handling of PwD matters. The Act describes welfare services for PwDs, emphasizing inclusion, rehabilitation, and capacity building, especially for minors and those in legal trouble. It aims to provide a just and inclusive society for PwDs (Wachira, 2021). Figure 2.1 compares disability-related laws in selected African and Asian countries.

2.4 Policy Implementation Challenges and Solutions

Turning a developed policy into a reality is known as policy implementation. It offers the operational domain for implementing the public policy announced by the appropriate authority. Integrating human, material, machine, and financial resources is essential in implementing public policy (Ajulor, 2018).

Improved public health and medical care have significantly reduced disabilities caused by malnutrition and infectious diseases. However, advancements in clinical treatment have also led to the survival of individuals with conditions that often result in long-term disabilities, such as congenital disabilities, injuries, diabetes, or HIV/AIDS. Additionally, the aging global population faces an increased risk of incapacitating conditions. Recognizing these challenges, initiatives like the "Global Grand Challenge of Disability and Development," introduced by the Obama White House, emphasize the necessity of interdisciplinary and global cooperation to create sustainable, disability-inclusive development strategies (Cogburn, 2017).

The main challenges in disability rehabilitation include understanding disability and accepting Community-Based Rehabilitation (CBR) as an effective intervention. Hospital-based services often lead to knowledge gaps, social isolation, and limited accessibility, benefiting fewer individuals. Effective use of resources, finance, human resources, and materials is essential, but poor planning, lack of coordination between sectors, and inadequate management of CBR services hinder progress. Other issues include insufficient evidence-based strategies, fragmented coordination between governments and NGOs, and a lack of coherent community-level approaches. Disability should be prioritized as a public health issue, with services integrated into mainstream development. A multi-sectoral approach covering social integration, health, education, and vocational programs is crucial. Primary healthcare should support early identification, essential interventions, and referrals to specialized services. Education must adapt to be more inclusive, while collaboration with employment sectors is needed to ensure access to training and work for PwDs. Monitoring and evaluation should be strengthened, focusing on outcomes like community mobilization, education, and employment opportunities. Additionally, service delivery, funding, and training research should be expanded, particularly for underserved populations in rural and small-town areas (Kumar et al., 2012).

Policy analysts highlight complexity as a significant barrier to effective policy implementation. It arises from multiple policy goals, leading to coordination challenges and resource dispersion across competing activities. Complexity also stems from the large number of actors and decision points involved, particularly in federal programs with implementation managed by regional offices and various state and local agencies. These agencies, often with differing objectives, must cooperate and coordinate to carry out federal agendas, complicating the implementation process (Percy, 1993).

The complexity challenges are exacerbated when different levels of government—federal, State, and local pursue their respective objectives without sufficient coordination. Policy implementation becomes fragmented when these entities have competing priorities, resources, and governance structures, making it difficult to achieve a unified approach to disability rehabilitation. Percy (1993) notes that such fragmentation leads to inefficiencies and often undermines the effectiveness of the overall policy. This requires better coordination across different government levels and the active involvement of community-based organizations and the private sector to ensure effective delivery of services.

The need for a cohesive and coordinated approach to disability rehabilitation becomes even more evident when considering the challenges faced by rural and underserved populations. In these areas, there is often a dearth of access to specialized healthcare services, educational resources, and employment opportunities for PwDs. This highlights the importance of developing localized solutions considering these populations' specific needs and contexts while aligning with national policies and frameworks (Kumar et al., 2012). Additionally, strengthening the capacity of local governments to manage and deliver disability-inclusive services and improving intersectoral collaboration can help overcome the barriers posed by rural and remote areas.

Promoting improved education by integrating employability and job skills into high school curricula is a policy solution that addresses the barriers, such as the late start to the "concept of work" and the broader societal stigma. Expanding employment opportunities was also a key policy solution (Khayatzadeh-Mahani et al., 2020). Vocational rehabilitation services should support both employers and employees. Employees may require assessments of their professional suitability and occupational preferences and services to improve their work performance, such as (re)training, increased awareness of available job opportunities, and skills training. Additionally, employees may need guidance on maintaining their health in the workplace. On the other hand, employers need information about the abilities and needs of PwDs, along with advice on making the work environment more accessible and supportive. Much of the success depends on the attitudes and efforts of employers, who can make a difference by adjusting the physical work environment often more quickly and affordably than they expect, offering flexible work arrangements, and fostering a supportive workplace culture (Hanga et al., 2015).

Various approaches have been implemented to enhance vehicles and infrastructure. In Africa and India, mobility solutions are primarily limited to small-scale pilot projects that explore different accessible service options and ad hoc infrastructure features or mobility aids provided by the private or welfare sectors. Broader improvements to transport systems focus on making them more user-friendly for all passengers, including those without disabilities. Efforts include improving the interfaces between passengers and the system and addressing challenges for individuals with visual, hearing, or cognitive impairments due to a lack of information. Additionally, there is a need to ensure access for people with severe physical disabilities, such as wheelchair users. Specialized door-to-door services are also being developed for passengers who cannot independently use any form of public transport (Venter et al., 2002).

Thus, the complexity of policy implementation in the disability sector demands a comprehensive, multi-layered approach that integrates resources, expertise, and efforts across various industries and levels of government. By prioritizing coordination, adopting evidence-based strategies, and fostering partnerships, it is possible to create a more inclusive and effective system for disability rehabilitation. This would improve the quality of life for PwDs and promote greater social and economic inclusion (Ajulor, 2018; Cogburn, 2017).

2.5 Conclusion

While significant strides have been made in establishing legal frameworks for disability rights across Asia and Africa, mirroring the progress seen in international conventions like the CRPD, substantial implementation gaps persist. The path toward achieving genuine inclusion for PwDs remains fraught with challenges, ranging from deeply ingrained societal stigma and inaccessible infrastructure to resource limitations and a lack of coordinated multi-sectoral approaches. Success hinges on strengthening legal frameworks, fostering inclusive education, accessible transportation and other essential services, promoting employment opportunities through vocational training and support, and actively engaging community-based rehabilitation initiatives. Addressing individual nations' unique cultural and socioeconomic contexts is crucial for developing effective and sustainable strategies. Continued advocacy, rigorous monitoring and evaluation of policies, and a commitment to evidence-based interventions are vital to bridging the gap between legal aspiration and lived reality for PwDs in these diverse and dynamic regions.

References

Ajulor, O. V. (2018). The challenges of policy implementation in Africa and sustainable development goals. *International Journal of Social Sciences, 3*(3), 1497–1518. https://doi.org/10.20319/pijss.2018.33.14971518

Akram, R., Buis, A., Sultana, M., Lauer, J. A., & Morton, A. (2024). Mapping gaps and exploring impairment and disability prevalence in South Asian (SAARC) countries: a scoping review. *Disability and Rehabilitation: Assistive Technology*, 1–14.

Balakrishnan, A., Kulkarni, K., Moirangthem, S., Kumar, C. N., Math, S. B., & Murthy, P. (2019). The rights of persons with disabilities Act 2016: Mental health implications. *Indian Journal of Psychological Medicine, 41*(2), 119–125. https://doi.org/10.4103/ijpsym.ijpsym_364_18

Bhattacharyya, R. (2014). Disability laws in India: A study. *International Journal of Research, 1*(4), 99–115.

Bruce, A., Quinn, G., Degener, T., Burke, C., Quinlivan, S., Castellino, J., Kenna, P., & Kilkelly, U. (2002). *Human rights and disability: The current use and future potential of United Nations human rights instruments in the context of disability*. United Nations Press.

Cannata, G., Douryang, M., Ljoka, C., Giordani, L., Monticone, M., & Foti, C. (2022). The burden of disability in Africa and Cameroon: a call for optimizing the education in physical and rehabilitation medicine. *Frontiers in Rehabilitation Sciences, 3*, 873362. https://doi.org/10.3389/fresc.2022.873362

Chou, Y. C., Uwano, T., Chen, B. W., Sarai, K., Nguyen, L. D., Chou, C. J., Mongkolsawadi, S., & Nguyen, T. T. (2024). Assessing disability rights in four Asian countries: The perspectives of disabled people on physical, attitudinal and cultural barriers. *Political Geography, 108*, 103027. https://doi.org/10.1016/j.polgeo.2023.103027

Cogburn, D. L. (2017, March). The grand challenge of disability and development in ASEAN. In D. L Cogburn & T. K. Reuter (Eds.), *Making disability rights real in Southeast Asia: Implementing the UN Convention on the rights of persons with disabilities in ASEAN*. Lexington Books.

Dube, A. K. (2005). The role and effectiveness of disability legislation in South Africa. *Samaita Consultancy and Programme Design*, 1–89.

References

ESCAP, U. (2023). Advancing SDG7 in Asia and the Pacific: policy briefs in support of the UN High-level political forum 2023.

Fernandez, E. L. A., Rutka, L. J., & Aldersey, H. M. (2017). Exploring disability policy in Africa: An online search for national disability policies and UNCRPD ratification. *Review of Disability Studies: An International Journal, 13*(1).

Gostin, L. O. (2000). Human rights of persons with mental disabilities: The European Convention of Human Rights. *International journal of law and psychiatry, 23*(2), 125–159.

Hanga, K., DiNitto, D. M., & Wilken, J. P. (2015). Promoting employment among people with disabilities: Challenges and solutions. *Social Work and Social Sciences Review, 18*(1), 31–51. https://doi.org/10.1921/swssr.v18i1.847

Hao, Y., & Li, P. (2020). Employment legal framework for persons with disabilities in china: Effectiveness and reasons. *International Journal of Environmental Research and Public Health, 17*(14), 4976. https://doi.org/10.3390/ijerph17144976

Haque, M. (2020). Disability brief in single chapter and Bangladesh perspectives: A rapid overview. *Advances in Human Biology, 10*(2), 41–50. https://doi.org/10.4103/AIHB.AIHB_6_20

Harpur, P. (2012). Embracing the new disability rights paradigm: The importance of the convention on the rights of persons with disabilities. *Disability & Society, 27*(1), 1–14. https://doi.org/10.1080/09687599.2012.631794

Hartley, M. T., & Tarvydas, V. M. (Eds.). (2022). *The professional practice of rehabilitation counseling*. Springer Publishing Company. https://doi.org/10.1891/9780826139047

Hughes, B. (2009). Disability activisms: Social model stalwarts and biological citizens. *Disability & Society, 24*(6), 677–688. https://doi.org/10.1080/09687590903160118

Islam, M. A., & Juhara, S. F. (2021). Rights and protection of persons with disabilities in Bangladesh: A critical review. *International Journal of Research and Innovation in Social Science, 5*(01), 331–335. https://doi.org/10.47772/IJRISS.2021.5114

Islam, M. Z., & Jahan, A. (2018). Disability rights: Challenges and opportunities in Bangladesh. *Journal of Asian and African Social Science and Humanities, 4*(2), 45–51.

Jagadeesan, A. J., Murugesan, R., Devi, S. V., Meera, M., Madhumala, G., Padmaja, M. V., Ramesh, A., Banerjee, A., Sushmitha, S., Khokhlov, A. N., & Marotta, F. (2017). Current trends in etiology, prognosis and therapeutic aspects of Parkinson's disease: A review. *Acta Bio Medica: Atenei Parmensis, 88*(3), 249. https://doi.org/10.23750/abm.v%vi%i.6063

Khayatzadeh-Mahani, A., Wittevrongel, K., Nicholas, D. B., & Zwicker, J. D. (2020). Prioritizing barriers and solutions to improve employment for persons with developmental disabilities. *Disability and Rehabilitation, 42*(19), 2696–2706. https://doi.org/10.1080/09638288.2019.1570356

Kumar, S. G., Roy, G., & Kar, S. S. (2012). Disability and rehabilitation services in India: Issues and challenges. *Journal of Family Medicine and Primary Care, 1*(1), 69–73. https://doi.org/10.4103/2249-4863.94458

Lang, R. (2009). The United Nations Convention on the right and dignities for persons with disability: A panacea for ending disability discrimination? *Alter, 3*(3), 266–285. https://doi.org/10.1016/j.alter.2009.04.001

Leshota, L. P. (2013). Reading the national disability and rehabilitation policy in the light of Foucault's technologies of power. *African Journal of Disability, 2*(1), 1–7. https://doi.org/10.4102/ajod.v2i1.41

Lord, J., & Stein, M. A. (2013). Prospects and practices for CRPD implementation in Africa. *Afr. Disability Rts. YB, 1*, 97.

Maja, P. A., Mann, W. M., Sing, D., Steyn, A. J., & Naidoo, P. (2011). Employing people with disabilities in South Africa. *South African Journal of Occupational Therapy, 41*(1), 24–32.

Math, S. B., Murthy, P., & Chandrashekar, C. R. (2011). Mental health act (1987): Need for a paradigm shift from custodial to community care. *Indian Journal of Medical Research, 133*(3), 246–249.

Mayhew, L. (2003). Disability—Global trends and international perspectives. *Innovation: The European Journal of Social Science Research, 16*(1), 3–28. https://doi.org/10.1080/135116103 04511

Meekosha, H., & Soldatic, K. (2011). Human rights and the global South: The case of disability. *Third World Quarterly, 32*(8), 1383–1397. https://doi.org/10.1080/01436597.2011.614800

Narayan, C. L., & John, T. (2017). The Rights of Persons with Disabilities Act, 2016: Does it address the needs of the persons with mental illness and their families. *Indian Journal of Psychiatry, 59*(1), 17–20. https://doi.org/10.4103/psychiatry.IndianJPsychiatry_75_17.

Neety, M. K. (2023). The right to education and employment for person with disabilities: Overview of Bangladesh perspective.

Nigussie Koski, A. (2021). *The voice of the invisible minority: An intersectional analysis of the integration of immigrants with disabilities in Finland* (Master's thesis). http://urn.fi/URN:NBN:fi:jyu-202106183908

Nuri, R. P., Aldersey, H. M., Ghahari, S., Huque, A. S., & Shabnam, J. (2022). The Bangladeshi Rights and Protection of Persons with Disability Act of 2013: A policy analysis. *Journal of Disability Policy Studies, 33*(3), 178–187. https://doi.org/10.1177/10442073211066789

Onazi, O. (2024). Duties of persons with disabilities under the African disability rights protocol: a sceptical argument. *Human Rights Law Review, 25*(2), ngaf004.

Onyango, G. O. (2012). *A socio-legal critique of the legal framework for the promotion of rights of persons with disabilities in Kenya*. Erasmus University of Rotterdam.

Parker, K. (2001). Changing attitudes towards persons with disabilities in Asia. *Disability Studies Quarterly, 21*(4). https://doi.org/10.18061/dsq.v21i4.322

Patterson, D. (2024). Human Rights-based Approaches and the Right to Health: A Systematic Literature Review. *Journal of Human Rights Practice, 16*(2), 603–623.

Percy, S. L. (1993, April). Challenges and dilemmas in implementing disability rights policies. *Journal of Disability Policy Studies., 4*(1), 41–63. https://doi.org/10.1177/104420739300400103

Pityana, B. (2003). The promotion of equality and prevention of unfair discrimination act 4 of 2000. *Codicillus, 44*(1), 2–9.

Rioux, M. H. (2011). Disability rights and change in a global perspective. *Sport in Society, 14*(9), 1094–1098. https://doi.org/10.1080/17430437.2011.614766

Sabatello, M., & Schulz, M. (2014). A short history of the international disability rights movement. *Human Rights and Disability Advocacy*, 13–24. https://doi.org/10.9783/978081220874 0.13

Stein, M. A., & Lord, J. E. (2021). A human rights perspective on disability-inclusive development. *Critical Issues in Human Rights and Development*, 86–106. https://doi.org/10.4337/978 1781005972.00012

Thabethe, W. (2022). An investigation of the implementation of the Employment Equity Act (No. 55 of 1998) of South Africa by organisations in Cape Town in the Western Cape.

Thongkuay, S. (2009). *Rights of persons with disabilities in the Asia Pacific*. Asia Pacific Human Rights Information Center. http://www.hurights.or.jp/ [11 April 2017].

UNESCAP. (2022). Framework for disability policies and strategies in Asia and the Pacific.

Union, A. (2015). Agenda2063 report of the commission on the African Union Agenda 2063 The Africa we want in 2063.

Vaughn, J. (2003). *Disabled rights: American disability policy and the fight for equality*. Washington, DC: Georgetown University Press.

Venter, C. J., Bogopane, H., Rickert, T., Camba, J., Venkatesh, A., Mulikita, N., Maunder, D., Savill, T., & Stone, J. (2002). Improving accessibility for people with disabilities in urban areas. *Proceedings: CODATU X. Lome*.

Wachira, A. (2021). *Access to justice for persons with disability in Kenya: Interrogating the adequacy of the legal framework* (Doctoral dissertation, University of Nairobi).

Walsham, M., Kuper, H., Banks, L. M., & Blanchet, K. (2019). Social protection for people with disabilities in Africa and Asia: A review of programmes for low-and middle-income countries. *Oxford Development Studies, 47*(1), 97–112. https://doi.org/10.1080/13600818.2018.1515903

Chapter 3
Socioeconomic Challenges Faced by People with Disabilities in Asia and Africa

Abstract This chapter examines the significant socioeconomic challenges faced by PwD in Asia and Africa. PwD in these regions experience disproportionately substantial poverty levels of poverty, scarce access to exceptional learning and healthcare, and insufficient social services. Systemic barriers, including physical inaccessibility, lack of trained personnel, societal stigma, and inadequate policy implementation, hinder their social inclusion and economic participation. The chapter explores the complex interplay between disability and poverty, highlighting the vicious cycle where poverty can lead to disability, and disability exacerbates poverty. It analyzes challenges in accessing education and quality services, workforce inclusion and economic empowerment, healthcare and rehabilitation, and strategies for breaking the link between disability and poverty. The chapter emphasizes the need for comprehensive policies and actions grounded in the principles of the UN CRPD to ensure the thorough partaking of PwDs in society.

Keywords Disability · Socioeconomic challenges · Poverty cycle · Disability stigma · And policy implementation

3.1 Introduction

Persons with disabilities (PwD) face significant socioeconomic challenges worldwide, particularly in Asia and Africa. These challenges are exacerbated by systemic barriers that limit access to education and quality services, essential for achieving social inclusion and economic participation. Globally, around one billion people, or approximately 15% of the population, live with some configuration of impairment, with a higher prevalence observed in developing regions, especially in Asia and Africa (Rohwerder, 2015). This demographic is disproportionately affected by poverty, limited healthcare access, and educational disparities. In Sub-Saharan Africa, PwD constitutes a significant portion of the impoverished population, with estimates suggesting that about 20% of people with low incomes are disabled (Sedeto & Dar, 2019).

Access to education is an entitlement human right enshrined in various international conventions. However, PwD often faces numerous barriers that prevent them from exercising this right. Physical accessibility is a major issue, with many educational institutions lacking the necessary infrastructure to accommodate students with physical disabilities. These institutions may have inaccessible classrooms, restrooms, and transportation options. Additionally, schools often lack appropriate materials and trained personnel to support children with disabilities. For example, assistive technologies and specialized teaching methods are frequently unavailable or underfunded. Attitudinal barriers, such as societal stigma and discrimination against PwD, also play a significant role. This can result in bullying and exclusion from school activities, creating a hostile environment that discourages attendance and participation, ultimately affecting educational outcomes (Rieser, 2012).

Even when PwD can ably enroll in educational institutions, their education quality is often substandard. Many teachers are not satisfactorily trained to address the student's needs with disabilities, leading to ineffective teaching practices that fail to support diverse learning requirements. Standard curricula are frequently not adapted for students with disabilities, hindering their learning experiences and limiting their academic achievements. As a result, dropout rates among students with disabilities are considerably higher than for their peers without disabilities. Children with disabilities often leave school earlier due to unmet needs or a hostile educational environment (Lyra et al., 2023).

Healthcare access is another critical area where PwD faces significant challenges. Healthcare facilities often lack necessary adaptations for individuals with mobility impairments, making it difficult for them to receive care. The financial burden associated with healthcare services is another barrier, particularly in low-income settings with limited resources. This economic strain is further exacerbated by the additional costs of managing a disability. Additionally, healthcare providers may lack the training needed to effectively treat patients with disabilities, leading to inadequate care and adverse health outcomes (Gudlavalleti, 2018).

Social services designed to support PwD are often insufficient. Many regions lack comprehensive social support programs that address the specific needs of PwD, such as rehabilitation services and community support systems. While legal frameworks exist to protect the rights of PwD, their implementation is often inadequate. Advocacy groups argue that while policies may exist on paper, they usually fail to translate into meaningful action on the ground (Aguilar, 2017).

The relationship between disability and poverty creates a vicious cycle that is difficult to break. Poverty can lead to higher rates of disability due to factors like malnutrition and lack of access to healthcare during critical developmental periods. On the other hand, individuals with disabilities face higher unemployment rates and lower income levels due to systemic discrimination in hiring practices and lack of workplace accommodations. Cultural perceptions of disability play a decisive contribution in shaping societal attitudes and treatment of PwD. In many Asian and African cultures, disability is often viewed with stigma or as a mark of disgrace for families. This perception can lead to social isolation for PwD and their families and affect policy decisions regarding disability rights and resource allocation (Groce et al., 2011).

The United Nations Convention on the Rights of Persons with Disabilities (CRPD) offers a global framework for advancing the rights of PwDs. It emphasizes the importance of accessibility to education and services as fundamental human rights. While many countries have ratified the convention, local implementation remains inconsistent. Various African nations have made progress toward inclusive education but face significant challenges. For example, in Ethiopia, children with disabilities encounter systemic barriers to accessing quality education due to insufficient resources and societal stigma. However, efforts are underway at the governmental level to improve conditions through policy reforms aimed at enhancing educational access (Sedeto & Dar, 2019). Despite policies mandating inclusion for PwD in education and employment in Kenya, enforcement remains weak due to cultural attitudes and economic constraints families face (Oranga & Gaungying, 2019). These global challenges underline the urgent need for comprehensive policies and actions to break the cycle of disability and poverty and ensure that PwD can fully participate in society.

3.2 Availability of Education and Standard of Services

A significant issue in the disability sector is the limited access to education for both children and adults with disabilities. Education is a fundamental right for all, as emphasized in the Universal Declaration of Human Rights and reinforced by innumerable intercontinental agreements, highlighting the importance of addressing this concern. In numerous countries, there is a significant gap between the educational prospects offered to children with disabilities compared to those available to their non-disabled peers. The intent of triumphing Education for All (EFA) will remain out of reach unless this situation is dramatically changed (Lindqvist, 1999).

In 2000, the Dakar Framework for Action endorsed the World Declaration on Education for All (EFA), intending to ensure that every child has access to elementary education by 2015. The framework identified Inclusive Education (IE) as a core initiative to achieve this goal. The Salamanca Statement and Framework for Action, supported by 92 governments and 25 international organizations at the 1994 World Conference on Special Needs Education in Salamanca, Spain, highlighted that every child has distinct learning needs, pursuits, individualities, and proficiencies. It emphasized the importance of integrating children with special educational needs (SEN) into mainstream schools, which should be equipped to address these needs using child-centered teaching approaches. The Statement also highlighted that educational systems that recognize and accommodate the diverse needs and characteristics of children are most operative in contending with discrimination, fostering inclusive communities, and achieving education for all. Such systems offer quality education for most children, enhancing the overall effectiveness and cost-efficiency of the education system. The main concept of all-encompassing schools is that all children, regardless of their challenges or differences, should learn together as much as possible. These schools need to acknowledge and respond to the miscellaneous prerequisites of their students, adjusting to dissimilar learning paces and styles. They should ensure quality education for all by offering appropriate curricula, teaching strategies, organizational arrangements, resources, and community partnerships. Each school should offer a variety of support and services to meet the diverse special needs of its students (Peter, 2004).

To live in this cutthroat environment, one needs to have the right information and abilities. People can get the skills and information they need to deal with the complexity of the world by having access to high-quality education (Peter, 2004; Ajita, 2013). Therefore, the importance of education for the progress of both entities and the nation as a whole is undeniable. Residents with higher levels of education are more aware of the difficulties facing their country and can make significant contributions to its advancement. In terms of health, edification empowers individuals to care for themselves and their families properly and make educated health decisions (Peter, 2004). For instance, educated women are more likely than illiterate women to seek prenatal care, assisted labor, and postnatal care, which lowers the risk of mother and infant mortality. As a result, education gives people the ability and opportunity to recognize and use their rights (Hulme, 2012).

PwDs typically have constrained connectivity to schools in many areas of the world, particularly in Asia and Africa, contempt for the value of education, and attempts to improve conscription (Uriah & Wosu, 2012). As an illustration, the United Nations Children's Fund (UNICEF) testified that, as of 2005, 67 million of the 200 million children with disabilities in the globe were not attending school. For nations in Africa, the situation can be worse (Hulme, 2012; Unicef, 2007). The World Health Organization reported that in 1997, just 0.3% of Ethiopia's 690,000 primary-aged children with disabilities were enrolled in school. In Rwanda, by 2001, only 300 out of 10,000 deaf children attended school, and in Burkina Faso, by 2006, only 10% of deaf children aged 7 to 12 were in school. A study report highlighted that in 1998, only 17% of the 30,000 disabled children in Lesotho were attending rudimentary education. While data on the educational outcomes of children with disabilities in Cameroon is limited, available information indicates that these children face significant educational barriers. For instance, a study by the International Centre for Evidence in Disability, 2014 in the North West Region of Cameroon found that children with disabilities were 20 times more likely to be unenrolled in school than their non-disabled peers (WHO, 2011).

Children with disabilities encounter numerous challenges that prevent them from accessing education. It has been highlighted that bodily accessibility to school buildings is crucial in ensuring education is available to children with impairments. Additional factors that limit enrollment and contribute to school dropouts among disabled children include incongruous teaching modus, unavailability of books, inadequately proficient teachers, insufficient schools, protracted distances to schools, and the high costs of educational materials such as books, pens, pencils, and textbooks. However, many academic institutions are designed without considering the prerequisites and apprehensions of PwDs, leading to this often-overlooked situation. Barriers that hinder children with physical or visual impairments from accessing education include

3.2 Availability of Education and Standard of Services

narrow doorways, impassable bathrooms, improper seating arrangements, uneven ground, and no ramps (Opoku et al., 2015).

The high unemployment and poverty rates among people with disabilities are primarily a result of their limited access to education, which has made it challenging for them to gain the essential dexterities requisite to vie with their non-disabled peers for employment in various segments of the economy (Brekke et al., 2023). International organizations and funding bodies have raised concerns about this issue and urged governments to give special focus to the education of children with impairments. For instance, Article 17 of the African Charter on Human and People's Rights emphasizes that everyone should have access to education (Filmer, 2008). Correspondingly, the UN Decade of Disabled Persons precedes the education and training of PwDs to ensure equivalent likelihoods for all members of society (UN, 1982) (African Charter on Human and Peoples Rights, 1981). Furthermore, Article 24 of the Convention on the Rights of Persons with Disabilities incites governments to convalesce educational opportunities for children with disabilities (United Nations International Children Emergency Fund promoting the Rights of Children with Disabilities, 2007). An ontogeny custom of research supports the principles (Peters, 2007) outlined in the Salamanca Statement. For instance, Metts (2000) references a 1993 World Bank study on Special Education in Asia, which clinched that 1) integrating primary school-aged children with Special Educational Needs (SEN) into widely held education that provides personal, social, and economic benefits; 2) most SEN can be effectively and more affordably supported in amalgamated schools rather than in parted institutional settings; and 3) the preponderance of children with SEN can be financially sustainable inclusion in primary schools (Metts, 2000).

Inclusive Education (IE) within the framework of Education for All (EFA) is a multifarious dispute, as disability spans multiple sectors, including employment, social welfare, education, and health (Cameron & Valentine, 2001). Consequently, developing policies for IE faces significant challenges, such as avoiding fragmented, unequal, and hard-to-avail services. IE can be applied at various levels, each with distinct goals, motivations, the cataloging of SEN, and service discernments. For instance, Kobi outlines six levels of IE: curricular, brute, psychological, civic, verbiage, and organizational (Abbring et al., 1995). The intent of IE may involve incorporating students with SEN into mainstream classrooms or transforming societal attitudes to promote better integration (Hornby, 2011). The objectives of IE may enhance educational outcomes and quality or encourage parental choice, consumer satisfaction, self-determination, and independence. However, the roundabouts of these objectives may skirmish with one another, creating tensions. Similarly, the reasons for adopting IE may arise from disgruntlement with the current system, concerns over pecuniary factors or resource distribution, or a desire for educational restructuring. Additionally, SEN services can be viewed in different ways: as a variety of placement alternatives (a multi-track model), as a distinct educational system (a two-track model), or as a spectrum of services within a single placement, such as in regular schools and classrooms (a one-track model) (European Agency for Development in Special Needs Education, 2003).

An additional stratum of convolution arises from how SEN are defined. Classification systems vary widely across different countries and even within countries. Some nations define special education needs based on the requirement for specialized services without labeling or quantifying students. For instance, the United Kingdom's 1978 Warnock Report delineated disability using this approach. Other countries adopt a two-tier classification, which considers both the type and severity of the disability and determines eligibility for special education based on educational underperformance and an "objective cause" of the disability. In these countries, disability categories differ. For instance, Denmark employs two categories, whereas Poland and the United States have over ten grades. However, most countries follow a categorical model, generally recognizing four to ten types of disabilities. In more outmoded societies, four primary sorts of disability are commonly acknowledged: intellectual disabilities, deafness, physical disability, and blindness. Additionally, some countries extend special education classifications to include non-disabled individuals, such as refugee children, gifted children, and those from marginalized groups who experience educational disadvantage, including street children, children from nomadic populations, or those affected by AIDS or civil unrest (Florian & McLaughlin, 2008).

The ISCED-97 (International Standard Classification of Education), espoused by OECD member countries, classifies students with SEN as those who receive extra public or private support to aid their education (Joint Research Centre, 2009). The resource-based definition includes students with an assortment of erudition challenges. The OECD further classifies these students into three groups based on the perceived causes of their educational challenges: Category A (students whose disabilities have clear biological origins), Category B (students with learning difficulties where no specific cause can be identified), and Category C (students facing challenges due to social disadvantages). There is increasing recognition that, for most students, the environment plays a key role in contributing to their disability.

The WHO's International Classification of Functioning and Disability (ICF) defines disability in two aspects: functioning and disability (covering body functions/structures and activities/participation), and contextual factors (which include environmental and personal elements). This approach shifts the perspective from viewing disability as an inherent deficiency to understanding it as the result of the interaction between the individual and their environment. It aligns with the social model of disability, which emphasizes the significance of environmental factors, as supported by disability rights groups and many individuals with disabilities (Peters, 2003). Ingstad (2001) contends that the distinctions made by the ICF are especially significant in many developing countries, where a person's identity is more closely tied to social roles and the fulfillment of family responsibilities than to individual capabilities.

The difference between impairment and impediment is fundamental. Disabled Persons International, 1981 defines impairment as the long-term or permanent reduction or loss of mental, sensory function, or physical. In contrast, disablement refers to the restriction or loss of opportunities to engage in customary community life due to brute and societal obstacles. The social construct of disability emphasizes environmental factors, proposing that societal obstacles primarily cause disability,

3.2 Availability of Education and Standard of Services

whereas the medical model views disability as an individual issue that requires medical treatment, therapy, or specialized care (Rieser, 2000).

The significant variation in the identification and categorization of children and young PwDs and SEN makes it challenging to assess the need for special education (Metts, 2000). A 1991 report by the Special Rapporteur on Human Rights and Disability found that at least 1 in 10 people in most countries have a mental, physical, or sensory impairment. Considering that these individuals are part of families, it is anticipated that disability impacts at least 25% of the population (Lansdown, 2001). Of the 500 million PwDs worldwide, 120–150 million are children, with 80% residing in developing countries. This number is expected to grow due to factors like rising poverty, armed conflicts, child labor, ferocity, abuse, and the HIV/AIDS epidemic. For example, the International Labour Organization (ILO) reports that of the 250 million children involved in labor, more than two–thirds (69%) are affected by injuries or illnesses, with around 15.6% (78 million) suffering impairments caused by accidents, distress, or warfare (Jerven, 2013).

In developing countries, 50% of disabilities are acquired before the age of 15, suggesting that the prevalence of disabled children and youth may be higher than the 10% incidence rate. The OECD estimates that 15–20% of all students will require special education during their primary and secondary school years (Kruk & Waśniewska, 2017). However, estimates of school attendance for children with disabilities in developing countries differ, with figures ranging from under 1% (Salamanca Framework for Action) to 5% (Peters et al., 2005). As a result, many children and young people with disabilities are denied educational opportunities at both the primary and secondary levels. The effectiveness and cost-efficiency of using categorical disability classifications are being challenged, as they may not adequately identify the services needed. To address barring and create tactics for incorporation, it is crucial to analyze policies and practices at three levels: micro-level (schools and communities), meso-level (educational systems and external organizations), and macro-level (national and international policy and legislation).

A study by Al Adawi et al. (2002) in Oman examined the stances of medical students and the accustomed public toward mental illness. The results showed no connection between attitudes and demographic factors such as personal experience, marital status, age (Akila et al., 2020), gender, or education with individuals living with mental illness. Both groups rejected genetic explanations for mental illness, instead attributing it to the influence of spirits. Participants generally had positive views on aspects such as the value of life, family relationships, decision-making abilities, and the care and management of mental illness. However, both medical students and the public tended to believe that individuals with mental illness often display unusual or stereotypical appearances, and most preferred psychiatric care facilities to be situated away from residential areas. A survey conducted in the United Arab Emirates found that only 38% of participants would seek help from mental health professionals if a family member, including their children, faced psychiatric issues. The main reasons for not seeking help included reluctance to accept that a family member had a mental illness, the stigma surrounding the use of mental health services, and doubts about their effectiveness. The likelihood of using psychiatric services was more significant among individuals with higher levels of parental education, better occupations, and a higher socioeconomic status (Eapen & Ghubash, 2004). Despite international efforts for inclusive education, children with disabilities face significant barriers to accessing education, especially in developing countries. These include physical inaccessibility, lack of resources, and societal stigma. Overcoming these challenges requires improving accessibility, teacher training, and inclusive policies. Only by addressing these issues can we ensure that education for all becomes a reality, empowering individuals with disabilities to contribute to society.

3.3 Workforce Inclusion and Economic Empowerment

PwD continues to experience significant disparities in economic inclusion globally. They face lower employment rates, earn considerably less, and are more likely to be employed in insecure jobs. These challenges are compounded by difficulties in obtaining workplace accommodations, especially for those with invisible or stigmatized disabilities, who often avoid disclosing their condition due to fear of discrimination. PwD also encounters more discrimination compared to their non-disabled peers. The intersection of these challenges with other forms of inequality, such as higher poverty rates and limited access to education, housing, transportation, healthcare, banking, and food, further exacerbates their economic exclusion. The COVID-19 pandemic has intensified these inequalities, with PwD experiencing job losses, reduced earnings, and difficulties accessing adequate social support. According to research, the pandemic exacerbated the disparities in job opportunities for people with and without disabilities and even within the disability community itself, highlighting the vulnerability of PwD during global crises (Blanck et al., 2024).

The United Nations' 2030 Agenda for Sustainable Development offers a comprehensive prototype for global serenity and opulence, emphasizing urgent action to reduce inequality, particularly for vulnerable groups like PwD. The Sustainable Development Goals (SDGs) specifically address disability-related issues, particularly regarding accessibility, employment, education, and equality. Figure 3.1 depicts the significant SDG goals mainly associated with disability.

Goal 8 seeks to achieve full and productive employment for everyone, including PwD, while Goal 10 is dedicated to reducing inequalities within and between countries. Despite these ambitious goals, inequality remains a pressing issue, with PwD continuing to face significant barriers to employment and equal opportunities in many countries (Suresh & Dyaram, 2020). Disability in India is a multifaceted issue deeply rooted in cultural narratives, with historical and social complexities. On one side, the major epics of India link disability to reduced perpetual childhood karma, evil, curses, and ability; on the other side, some representations depict disability as a symbol of strength and resilience in the struggle against oppression (Ghai, 2001).

Historically, PwD in India has been marginalized and excluded from mainstream development, with government policies contributing to this exclusion focusing

3.3 Workforce Inclusion and Economic Empowerment

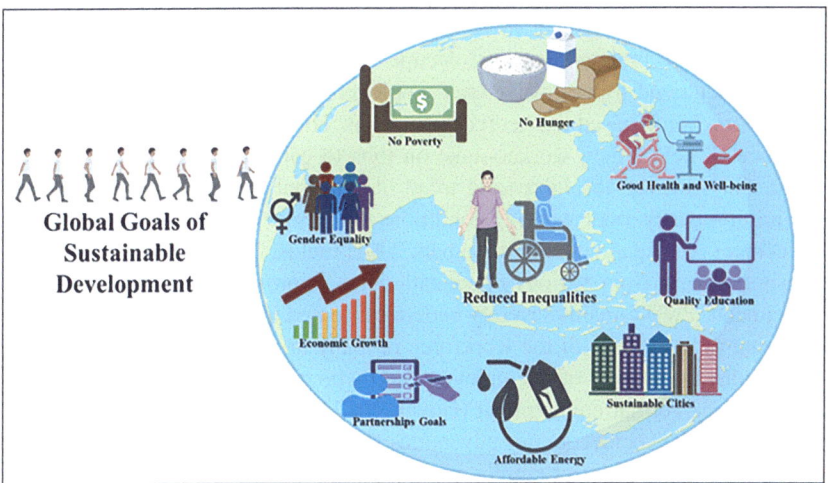

Fig. 3.1 Illustration of the global goals of sustainable development (This figure illustrates key Sustainable Development Goals (SDGs) to foster an inclusive and equitable society. The central theme, Reduced Inequalities, emphasizes the need for accessibility and equal opportunities for all, including persons with disabilities. These elements highlight the interconnected efforts required to promote a fair, sustainable, and inclusive world. The visual representation reinforces the importance of global collaboration in achieving these objectives)

mainly on protection and charity rather than empowerment. After India gained independence, disability policy remained centered around providing support for PwD to cope with daily challenges, reflecting an individual-focused approach (Kundu, 2000). In contemporary decades, India has experienced a momentous shift in the perception of disability and the rights of PwD, focusing on equalizing opportunities. A key turning point in this change was the introduction of the PwDs (Protection of Rights, Full Participation, and Equal Opportunities) Act in 1995, which aimed to provide greater rights and opportunities for PwDs. However, the Act faced criticism for adhering to the impairment-based model, focusing on particularized deficits rather than broader social inclusion (Ghosh, 2016; Mehrotra, 2011).

A significant shift occurred with the UN CRPD adoption in December 2006, which India ratified. This resulted in the depiction of the Rights of Persons with Disabilities (RPwD) Act in 2016, which replaced the earlier 1995 Act. The RPwD Act aligned with the UN CRPD, emphasizing a social and rights-based approach to disability, including equal employment opportunities, reservation in government jobs, and incentives for private-sector employers to promote inclusion. However, despite these legislative advances, statistical data reveals that PwD in India still experiences significantly fewer employment opportunities than the general population (Gudlavalleti et al., 2014; Mizunoya & Mitra, 2013). A substantial share of PwD is self-employed, with 36% engaged in work. Of these, 23% are cultivators, 31% are agricultural laborers, 4% work in household industries, and 42% are involved in other forms of employment (Ministry of Statistics and Programme Implementation, 2016). The preponderance of occupied PwDs is found in the unorganized sector, characterized by non-wage (self-employed) and wage-based (e.g., subcontract workers, home-based workers) employment. This sector is often viewed as an "easy-access" field where workers take on jobs to earn some income rather than none at all. However, the increasing trend of informal labor has raised concerns about job insecurity, poor working conditions, and limited opportunities for career advancement (Canagarajah & Sethuraman, 2001; Fields, 2004).

Despite efforts from various organizations to improve disability employment and inclusion, PwD remains severely underrepresented in the organized workforce, comprising only 1%–2% of the workforce in many organizations, a stark contrast to the significant number of unemployed PwD who continue to encounter difficulties in securing formal employment (Goyal, 2017; Shenoy, 2011). In Bangladesh, PwD faces similar socioeconomic adversities, confronted by significant poverty and constrained educational and employment opportunities. The country's per capita income in 2014 was just $1,088, and despite a reduction in poverty from 31.5% in 2010 to 24.3% in 2016, PwD remains one of the most disadvantaged groups. The exact prevalence of disability in Bangladesh is difficult to determine, with estimates ranging from 0.94% to 31.9%, reflecting significant underreporting and gaps in data collection. PwD in Bangladesh often face discrimination and lack opportunities in education and formal labor markets, with limited legislative action and poor enforcement of disability quotas in employment. Gender disparities are also pronounced, as women with disabilities face compounded discrimination based on both gender and disability, which severely limits their access to education and employment (Razzaque & Hasan, 2024).

In Kenya, a lower-middle-income country with a predominantly rural population, the inclusion of PwD in the workforce is hindered by distinct economic challenges. Approximately 20.9% of the population lives in extreme poverty, and underemployment is a more significant concern than outright unemployment, as 83% of the workforce is engaged in the informal sector, where decent work opportunities are scarce. Although Kenya has a more established legal framework for disability rights, including a 5% employment quota for PwD in both the public and private sectors, these policies have had limited success in improving actual employment outcomes for PwD. Despite progressive policies, only about 1% of PwD are employed in formal jobs. Employers often hold misconceptions about the capabilities of PwD, and social stigma remains widespread, with women with disabilities facing additional barriers such as gender-based discrimination and restricted educational opportunities. These determinants contribute to the significant underrepresentation of PwD in stable, formal employment opportunities in Kenya (Wickenden et al., 2020).

In Nigeria, a diverse and multi-ethnic country with a population of over 182 million people, PwD faces significant barriers to employment due to societal discrimination, inadequate infrastructure, and negative attitudes toward disability. Although the country has made some progress in addressing disability issues, over half of the population lives in multidimensional poverty, with many PwD experiencing reduced access to education, training, and job opportunities. Many disabled individuals also face challenges due to poor public transport and inaccessible buildings, further hindering their ability to participate in the workforce. Women with disabilities in Nigeria face additional challenges due to societal norms, which often exclude them from education and employment. The disability movement in Nigeria is fragmented, with many organizations still adhering to a benevolent approach instead of a rights-based strategy. National organizations like the Joint National Association of PwD (JONAPwD) and ASCEND advocate for the rights of PwD, but the lack of unity and strategic planning remains a significant challenge. Despite some efforts, such as vocational training programs and small loans aimed at promoting entrepreneurship, the effectiveness of these initiatives remains uncertain (Angell et al., 2022).

Uganda, with a predominantly rural population, faces high poverty rates and limited formal job opportunities, particularly for PwD. Most employment is in the informal sector, and despite some growth in formal sector waged jobs, poverty remains high, particularly among PwD. People with disabilities in Uganda make up only 1.3% of the formal workforce, often relegated to low-paying, precarious jobs. They face significant barriers to employment, including stigma, discrimination, and a lack of reasonable accommodations. While Uganda has relatively strong disability-inclusive policies, the implementation of these policies remains weak. Partnerships between organizations like the National Union of Disabled Persons of Uganda (NUDIPU), the Federation of Uganda Employers (FUE), and international NGOs work to raise awareness and create job opportunities. However, employer reluctance to adopt inclusive practices, as well as limited awareness and accessible information, continue to make it difficult for PwD to secure formal, stable employment (Wickenden et al., 2020).

In Asia and Africa, PwD faces significant barriers to economic inclusion, including inadequate enforcement of legal frameworks, societal stigma, and limited access to education and formal employment. While countries like India and Bangladesh have made strides with legislation aimed at promoting disability rights, PwD remains marginalized mainly, often working in the informal sector with limited job security. Similarly, in Kenya, Nigeria, and Uganda, despite existing disability-inclusive policies and employment quotas, PwD still encounters discrimination, poor infrastructure, and a lack of opportunities, especially for women with disabilities. Both regions share common challenges but require more substantial implementation of policies, greater awareness, and improved access to education and formal employment to include PwD in the workforce.

3.4 Healthcare and Rehabilitation: Gaps in Accessibility

PwDs, especially in less economically developed countries, encounter substantial impediments to retrieving healthcare amenities and support, exacerbated during disasters and emergencies. During the COVID-19 pandemic, for instance, many people with disabilities struggled to access healthcare facilities, treatments, rehabilitation, and necessary medications. Even those who could reach healthcare facilities often faced difficulties, including direct discrimination when seeking critical care such as intensive care unit (ICU) admission or ventilator support. Additionally, research indicates that PwDs are at a higher menace of contracting the virus due to factors such as their reliance on personal caregivers and their residence in group settings or residential facilities (McKinney et al., 2021).

Providing optimal rehabilitation services to people with disabilities is a critical concern for health systems worldwide. Despite differences in the organization, financing, and delivery of healthcare, all countries face similar challenges. For example, one key challenge in Iran is trusteeship, with the Ministry of Health overseeing healthcare and establishing the General Department of Rehabilitation in 2014. The Red Crescent Organization also stipulates independent rehabilitation services. Since 1980, the Welfare Organization has been responsible for rehabilitation services, but in 2014, the Supreme Leader's health policies placed the Ministry of Health accountable for organizing and overseeing rehabilitation services. However, financing remains a significant challenge, especially in economically underprivileged countries, as it impacts the overall functioning of the health system. Additionally, Iran faces a shortage of specialized personnel and rehabilitation centers, which is exacerbating the situation. Considering the country's political and economic circumstances and the growing population of individuals with disabilities, there is an urgent need for a coordinated and efficient system for providing rehabilitation services to address these challenges (Iravani et al., 2021).

PwDs in South Asia face the exact customary health needs of others and additional healthcare challenges. They require treatment for ordinary circumstances like viral fevers, malaria, respiratory infections, and diarrhea. In addition to these general health requirements, individuals also need assistive devices or treatment for their underlying impairments, such as polio, cleft palate, intellectual disabilities, and learning difficulties. Moreover, people with disabilities face a higher likelihood of coexisting conditions, particularly non-communicable diseases, and generally require more frequent counseling compared to those without disabilities. Studies from South Asia and other developing countries also highlight these needs. LMICS indicates that people with disabilities bear a heavier health burden, often resulting in more extended hospital stays, frequent hospital readmissions, and increased medication requirements (Murthy et al., 2014). For example, in Bangladesh, 85% of individuals with physical disabilities affirmed experiencing a general illness within the past six months. Despite these heightened health risks, their access to healthcare services is frequently obstructed by factors outside their control, affecting all healthcare system levels, from primary care to tertiary facilities.

The CRPD mandates that states ensure equal healthcare access for PwDs. Article 25 of the CRPD particularly underscores health as a right, guaranteeing equivalent access to the best possible level of health for PwDs and obligating governments to adjust healthcare services to address their unique needs. The Sustainable Development Goals (SDGs) also emphasize the inclusion of PwDs as essential for achieving sustainable development and highlight the requisite to enhance healthcare access for everyone through Universal Health Coverage (UHC), which must encompass people with disabilities. Experts contend that if healthcare programs fail to reach individuals with disabilities, it signifies the ineffectiveness of these initiatives. For instance, an appraisal of two representative household surveys in Afghanistan, conducted in 2005 and 2013, divulged that the perceived accessibility of healthcare and satisfaction with healthcare reportage significantly declined for people with disabilities over that period, contempt of the existence of an unpretentious health service package for all. Prioritizing the health prerequisites of persons with disabilities: Inclusive health encompasses all aspects of healthcare, from policies to service delivery, and is grounded in affordability, equity, and efficacy. Inclusive health goes beyond merely providing healthcare services; it involves taking proactive measures to ensure that PwDs, along with other marginalized and discriminated groups, have access to the necessary healthcare. This approach authorizes them to bestow the development of their communities actively. Public health should prioritize meeting the evolving health needs of all populations, including individuals with disabilities. Collaborating with all stakeholders, including PwDs, is essential for reducing poor health, promoting overall well-being, and enhancing eminence of life. It ensures that PwDs are integrated into society and not excluded due to their health conditions (Gudlavalleti, 2018).

The United Nations Enable Newsletter, 2014 (http://www.un.org/disabilities) reports that people with disabilities globally experience poorer health outcomes and are more likely to encounter barriers in accessing healthcare compared to non-disabled individuals. PwDs are twice as likely to find healthcare providers meager, three times more likely to be repudiated care, and four times more likely to face mistreatment. Research by Lishner et al. (1996) emphasized that although individuals in rural areas face challenges accessing primary healthcare, these difficulties are exacerbated for PwDs. The EquitAble Project 2011 examined healthcare access issues for PwDs in impoverished settings, including South Africa, Malawi, Namibia, and Sudan. It found that structural barriers such as transport, facility accessibility, long waiting times, and cost hindered access to care, alongside issues like inadequate communication, negative attitudes from healthcare workers, and a lack of trained personnel.

Moreover, individuals with disabilities are more prone to health issues related to both communicable diseases (such as TB, HIV, and malaria) and non-communicable diseases (including cancer, cardiovascular conditions, and diabetes). Similar obstacles to PwDs accessing healthcare have been identified in developed and developing nations. Research in developed countries indicates that PwDs face higher rates of illness and hospitalization, with barriers to access arising from factors like cost, transportation, and the need for assistance from attendants. In Africa, the EquitAble project found that transport, cost, and distance were significant obstacles to healthcare access for people with disabilities. Poverty further complicates this issue, as poor individuals with disabilities face added challenges such as lack of awareness, inaccessible facilities, financial constraints, and inadequate transport. A rural South African study revealed that multiple factors, including these barriers, interact to limit healthcare access, worsening existing health conditions and increasing the risk of preventable health issues. Moreover, different types of disabilities, such as hearing or mobility impairments, present unique access needs, such as sign language interpreters or properly prescribed wheelchairs. Ultimately, inadequate access to healthcare can exacerbate health outcomes for people with disabilities. Understanding these healthcare needs and the barriers that people with disabilities face is essential to improving both general and specialized healthcare services. While studies comparing health outcomes and access to healthcare services for PwDs are available globally and within the African region, there is a shortage of thorough comparative research on this matter, specifically within South Africa (Moodley & Ross, 2015).

In both South Asia and Africa, people with disabilities encounter significant barriers to accessing healthcare, though the nature of these challenges varies by region. In South Asia, key gaps in accessibility include inadequate healthcare infrastructure, limited rehabilitation services, and a lack of specialized healthcare professionals, all of which contribute to poor health sequels for PwDs. Additionally, individuals with disabilities in this region face an increased menace of co-morbid occurrences such as non-communicable diseases, which further complicate their ability to access healthcare. Similarly, in Africa, the primary barriers to healthcare include transport issues, high costs, and the physical inaccessibility of healthcare facilities. Rural areas in both regions face additional challenges, such as long distances to healthcare centers and insufficient financial resources.

Furthermore, people with disabilities in both regions experience discrimination, negative attitudes from healthcare providers, and a lack of accommodations, such as sign language interpreters or mobility aids, which further exacerbate their exclusion from quality care. Although both regions recognize the importance of inclusive healthcare through international frameworks like the CRPD and SDGs, structural gaps remain in policy implementation, specialized services, and funding. Addressing these gaps is crucial to improving healthcare accessibility, ensuring that people with disabilities are not marginalized, and achieving universal health coverage and sustainable development in both regions.

3.5 Breaking the Link Between Disability and Poverty

Focusing too narrowly on specific diseases can overshadow the ongoing and significant issue of "diseases of poverty," which remains a major driver of disability, particularly in low-income areas. In the "Consultations with the Poor" study, illness was seen as a direct consequence of poverty in seven out of nine villages in Malawi. In comparison, only two villages viewed illness as a cause of poverty. This highlights the cyclical relationship between poverty and disability, where poor living conditions, lack of access to healthcare, and inadequate sanitation contribute to illness. In turn, disability worsens a family's financial situation. Acton emphasizes that untreated impairments can push families further into poverty, with the loss of income due to disability exacerbating financial instability (Elwan, 1999).

Poverty itself can create or intensify disabilities, as poor access to nutrition, healthcare, and preventive measures can lead to physical and mental impairments. This relationship is often underappreciated in policy discussions but requires urgent attention to break the cycle. Research identifies three primary ways disability worsens a family's financial situation: (1) Loss of Income, where disabled individuals or their caregivers are unable to work, reducing the family's income; (2) Additional Costs, including medical expenses, assistive devices, and care for people with disabilities, which drain family resources; and (3) Marginalization and Exclusion, as disabled individuals often face barriers to essential services and social activities, deepening their economic vulnerability. Furthermore, certain groups, such as women, children, and those in rural areas, are more vulnerable to these economic challenges, facing both social and geographical hindrances that further impede their access to education, employment, and healthcare. As a result, PwDs not only suffer from physical impairments but also from a compounded economic disadvantage that is hard to overcome. A comprehensive approach is needed to break this cycle, including access to affordable healthcare, inclusive education, employment opportunities, and support for caregivers. Only by addressing both the immediate needs for healthcare and the broader social and economic barriers can we hope to support disabled individuals in overcoming the long-term financial and social challenges they face (Elwan, 1999).

Much of the discussion about the financial impact of disability on individuals and their families has historically focused on developed countries, often in the context of analyzing various compensation and assistance schemes. Regardless of the country, the costs generally include direct expenses related to the disability and costs incurred by those providing care, in addition to the lower incomes of disabled individuals. The direct costs of disability may involve medical expenses, assistive devices (like crutches or wheelchairs), specialized services, and home modifications, all of which can be considerable. A recent survey of disabled people in India found that the direct costs for treatment and equipment ranged from the equivalent of three days' income to two years' income, with the average cost amounting to about two months' worth of income (Peprah et al., 2023). Table 3.1 illustrates the key challenges and aspects of inclusive education for PwDs across different regions.

The costs of providing care for a disabled person may be borne in different ways: some may be directly covered by the individual, others may be met by state or local authorities through welfare systems, and some are borne by friends or family members providing care. The 1980s Summary Declaration Charter highlighted that approximately 25% of people in a community are hindered from fully expressing their capacities due to disability, including not just the disabled individuals but also their families and those who assist them. Additionally, the financial strain on caregivers, especially the loss of employment and income, has gained increasing recognition. The impact on the standard of living for other family members due to the caregiver's loss of earnings further exacerbates financial challenges. These costs underline the multifaceted financial burden faced by disabled individuals and their families, impacting not just medical expenses but also daily living and long-term stability (Callahan et al., 1980).

Table 3.1 Key challenges and aspects of inclusive education for PwDs across different regions

Region/Area	Key challenges	Main aspects
Global	Limited access to education for children with disabilities, especially in developing countries	Education is a basic human right
	Lack of specialized resources, teacher training, and inclusive policies	International frameworks like the Universal Declaration of Human Rights and the Salamanca Statement support inclusive education
	High unemployment and poverty rates due to limited educational opportunities	Inclusive Education (IE) aims to integrate children with disabilities into mainstream schools with appropriate support systems
Asia (e.g., India, China, etc.)	Inadequate infrastructure, including lack of ramps, narrow doorways, and inaccessible school facilities	A large population of PwDs face significant barriers to access
	Insufficient special education services and trained teachers	In Asia, children with disabilities are often excluded from mainstream education
	Stigma and societal attitudes toward disabilities	Some countries have developed specific policies to improve access, but challenges remain in rural and underserved areas
Africa (e.g., Ethiopia, Rwanda)	Low enrollment rates for children with disabilities, with examples like Ethiopia (0.3% of children with disabilities in school)	A significant portion of children with disabilities are excluded from education (e.g., 67 million children globally do not attend)
	Physical inaccessibility of schools and lack of specialized services	Many children face high rates of dropout due to physical barriers and lack of proper accommodations in schools
	Limited awareness and societal stigma	International efforts (e.g., UNICEF and WHO reports) highlight the severity of educational exclusion in Africa
Europe (e.g., UK, Denmark)	Disparities in educational services and classification systems for disabilities	Some countries use a categorical model to classify disabilities; others focus on needs-based definitions
	Limited understanding of inclusive education in certain countries	Policies like the Warnock Report in the UK have shaped inclusive education but still face implementation challenges

(continued)

3.5 Breaking the Link Between Disability and Poverty

Table 3.1 (continued)

Region/Area	Key challenges	Main aspects
	Need for integration of PwDs in general education settings rather than segregated systems	Efforts to promote awareness and integrate children with disabilities into mainstream schools have led to varying success
Middle East (e.g., UAE, Oman)	Negative cultural attitudes and stigma surrounding disability	Medical model views of disability are prevalent, which can limit opportunities for inclusive education
	Societal reluctance to accept mental health issues limits access to education for those with cognitive disabilities	Surveys show that people prefer psychiatric facilities away from residential areas, reflecting the stigma surrounding disabilities
	Insufficient teacher training and resources for inclusive education	Need for a shift in societal perceptions toward more inclusive practices and attitudes
Latin America (e.g., Brazil)	Societal exclusion and lack of public awareness regarding the rights of PwDs	Educational reform is ongoing, with increased attention on inclusive education, but challenges remain in rural and impoverished areas
	Limited funding for the integration of children with disabilities in mainstream schools	International standards, such as the UN Convention on the Rights of Persons with Disabilities, are being incorporated into policies
Caribbean (e.g., Jamaica, Haiti)	Lack of infrastructure, especially in rural areas, to accommodate children with physical disabilities	Educational systems increasingly adopt inclusive education models but still lack universal access to PwDs
	Social stigma, which results in underreporting and lack of support for children with disabilities	Some countries have made progress by integrating inclusive education policies but must tackle the remaining barriers

In Africa and Asia, research on disability's socioeconomic impact is limited but suggests individuals with disabilities face lower social and economic status, similar to patterns observed globally. Research consistently indicates that children with disabilities are less likely to begin or partake in school. For instance, research in African countries like Malawi, Rwanda, and Zambia and Asian nations like India and Cambodia indicates lower school enrollment rates among children with disabilities. In terms of adult education, individuals with disabilities in these regions generally have lower educational attainment, although a study in urban Sierra Leone found no such effect. Healthcare access is another challenge; studies in India and Sierra Leone show reduced access to healthcare for people with disabilities, often accompanied by higher healthcare spending. Economic disparities are also evident. Households with disabilities in both Africa (e.g., Malawi, Zambia, and Mozambique) and Asia (e.g., India) tend to own fewer assets, face lower incomes, and have fewer household expenditures compared to non-disabled households. However, results vary across countries, with some studies showing no significant differences. Living conditions are typically worse for families with disabilities in countries like Namibia and Mozambique. Cross-country studies in these regions find that disability is often associated with higher poverty rates, but the relationship weakens when factors like education are accounted for. Therefore, the evidence in both Africa and Asia suggests that people with disabilities are economically disadvantaged, but the findings are not universally conclusive due to differences in study methodologies and disability definitions (Mitra et al., 2011).

Though various policies are being implemented for the betterment of people with disabilities, international initiatives, like the Vocational Rehabilitation and Employment Convention and the Standard Rules on the Equalization of Opportunities, have highlighted the need for policies supporting disabled people. While recognition of the need for policy change is growing, the ratification and implementation of these policies remain slow, with many challenges still to be addressed. The literature on disability policies differs significantly between developed and developing countries. In developed countries, the focus is on public programs, both governmental and privately regulated, to cover disability risks. These programs typically separate work-related disabilities from non-work-related ones, with some countries providing comprehensive rehabilitative services and targeting disability benefits to those fully incapacitated, aiming to promote employment. In middle-income countries, disability pensions are common, covering significant portions of the labor force, especially in Asia.

In many developing countries, especially low-income ones, public or employer-funded disability programs are unavailable for those in the informal labor market. PwDs in rural and informal sectors often depend on family support, as state-provided services are scarce. Volunteer organizations may offer limited services, but these tend to be small-scale and sector-specific (Hendriks, 2007). In countries where communicable diseases and malnutrition often cause disability, prevention is crucial. Research in India, for example, found a widespread need for basic assistive equipment, such as glasses and crutches. Many people with visual impairments had no access to treatment, particularly in rural areas.

There is growing recognition that specialized, ad hoc services are insufficient in poorer communities. This has led to a shift from institutionalization toward more community-based approaches, like Community-Based Rehabilitation (CBR), which involve self-reliant schemes and participatory methods. Examples include CBR programs for disabled refugees in Kenya and slum dwellers in other regions. Disabled individuals increasingly advocate for greater inclusion in mainstream workplaces and educational systems. The shift toward inclusive schooling, where children with special needs are unified into regular schools, has shown that most can be accommodated cost-effectively without disadvantaging other students. However, further research and evaluation of these inclusive approaches are still needed (Elwan, 1999).

While both Asia and Africa share similar challenges related to the socioeconomic impact of disability, key differences exist in the access to services and the effectiveness of existing policies. In both regions, individuals with disabilities face significant economic disadvantages, including lower education levels, limited healthcare access, and increased poverty rates. However, the availability of disability-related support systems and social protection programs varies considerably. In many African and Asian countries, especially low-income areas, public disability programs are either underdeveloped or unavailable, leaving disabled individuals and their families to rely heavily on informal support networks. The situation is exacerbated by the lack of basic healthcare and rehabilitation services, particularly in rural areas. Moreover, while Asia has seen some success in the implementation of disability pensions and other formal support mechanisms, many African nations still struggle with limited infrastructure for disability support. However, both regions are increasingly embracing CBR and inclusive education, which offer promising alternatives to institutionalization and can help break the cycle of poverty and disability. Ultimately, both continents need a more inclusive, comprehensive approach that addresses both immediate needs and long-term socioeconomic barriers, emphasizing prevention, education, and employment opportunities for disabled individuals.

3.6 Conclusion

PwD in Asia and Africa face a complex web of interconnected socioeconomic challenges that perpetuate a cycle of poverty and exclusion. While legal frameworks like the UN CRPD and national policies exist, their practical implementation remains significantly hampered by systemic barriers. These barriers include physical inaccessibility of education and healthcare facilities, a lack of trained personnel, pervasive societal stigma and discrimination, and inadequate social support systems. The economic consequences are severe, with PwD experiencing higher unemployment rates, lower incomes, and greater reliance on the precarious informal sector. Breaking this cycle requires a multi-pronged approach prioritizing inclusive education, accessible healthcare and rehabilitation services, employment opportunities with reasonable accommodations, and a fundamental shift in societal attitudes toward disability. Investing in preventive measures to reduce the incidence of acquired disabilities, particularly in low-income settings, is also crucial. Ultimately, achieving true social inclusion and economic empowerment for PwDs demands strong political will, robust policy implementation, and active participation of PwDs themselves in the design and execution of effective interventions.

References

Abbring, I. M., Hegarty, S., Meijer, C. J., & Pijl, S. J. (Eds.). (1995). *New perspectives in special education: A six-country study of integration.* Routledge. https://doi.org/10.4324/9780203976289

African Charter on Human and Peoples Rights (1981).

Ajita, N. (2013). Importance of education for sustainable development. *World Wide Fund.*

Al-Adawi, S., Dorvlo, A. S., Al-Ismaily, S. S., Al-Ghafry, D. A., Al-Noobi, B. Z., Al-Salmi, A., ... & Chand, S. P. (2002). Perception of and attitude towards mental illness in Oman. *International journal of social psychiatry, 48*(4), 305–317. https://psycnet.apa.org/doi/https://doi.org/10.1177/0020764002128783334

Akila, K., Divya, R., Preethianushya, M., Aravindhan, B., & Rogina, J. S. (2020). Assessment of cognitive impairment among elderly in the selected rural community, Kancheepuram District, Tamil Nadu. *Indian Journal of Public Health Research & Development, 11*(3), 19–21. https://doi.org/10.37506/ijphrd.v11i3.599

Angell, B., Sanuade, O., Adetifa, I. M., Okeke, I. N., Adamu, A. L., Aliyu, M. H., ... & Abubakar, I. (2022). Population health outcomes in Nigeria compared with other west African countries, 1998–2019: A systematic analysis for the global burden of disease study. *The Lancet, 399*(10330), 1117–1129. https://doi.org/10.1016/S0140-6736(21)02722-7

Blanck, P., Hyseni, F., & Goodman, N. (2024). Economic inclusion and empowerment of people with disabilities. In Handbook of disability: critical thought and social change in a globalizing world (pp. 1207–1228). Springer Nature Singapore. https://doi.org/10.1007/978-981-19-6056-7_81

Brekke, I., Alecu, A., Ugreninov, E., Surén, P., & Evensen, M. (2023). Educational achievement among children with a disability: Do parental resources compensate for disadvantage? *SSM-Population Health, 23,* Article 101465. https://doi.org/10.1016/j.ssmph.2023.101465

Callahan, J. J., Jr., Diamond, L. D., Giele, J. Z., & Morris, R. (1980). Responsibility of families for their severely disabled elders. *Health Care Financing Review, 1*(3), 29.

Cameron, D., & Valentine, F. (Eds.). (2001). *Disability and federalism: Comparing different approaches to full participation* (Vol. 62). IIGR, Queen's University.

Canagarajah, S., & Sethuraman, S. V. (2001). *Social protection and the informal sector in developing countries: Challenges and opportunities.* World Bank.

Devandas Aguilar, C. (2017). Social protection and persons with disabilities. *International Social Security Review, 70*(4), 45–65. https://doi.org/10.1111/issr.12152

Eapen, V., & Ghubash, R. (2004). Help-seeking for mental health problems of children: Preferences and attitudes in the United Arab Emirates. *Psychological Reports, 94*(2), 663–667. https://doi.org/10.2466/pr0.94.2.663-667

Elwan, A. (1999). *Poverty and disability: A survey of the literature* (Vol. 9932, pp. 1–48). Washington, DC: Social Protection Advisory Service.

European Agency for Development in Special Needs Education. (2003). *Special Needs Education in Europe.* A Thematic Publication by EADSNE.

Fields, G. S. (2004). A guide to multisector labor market models.

Filmer, D. (2008). Disability, poverty, and schooling in developing countries: Results from 14 household surveys. *The World Bank Economic Review, 22*(1), 141–163. https://doi.org/10.1093/wber/lhm021

Florian, L., & McLaughlin, M. J. (2008). *Disability classification in education: Issues and perspectives.* Corwin Press.

Ghai, A. (2001). *Marginalisation and disability: Experiences from the third world.* Disability and the life course: Global perspectives, 26. https://doi.org/10.1017/CBO9780511520914.005

Ghosh, N. (2016). Interrogating disability in India. *International Journal for Equity in Health, 19,* 131.

Goyal, M. (2017). Why companies are hiring people with disabilities?. *Economic Times.*

References

Groce, N., Kett, M., Lang, R., & Trani, J. F. (2011). Disability and poverty: The need for a more nuanced understanding of implications for development policy and practice. *Third World Quarterly, 32*(8), 1493–1513. https://doi.org/10.1080/01436597.2011.604520

Gudlavalleti, , M. V. S., John, N., Allagh, K., Sagar, J., Kamalakannan, S., Ramachandra, S. S., & South India Disability Evidence Study Group. (2014). Access to health care and employment status of people with disabilities in South India, the SIDE (South India Disability Evidence) study. *BMC Public Health, 14*, 1–8. https://doi.org/10.1186/1471-2458-14-1125

Gudlavalleti, V. S. M. (2018). Challenges in accessing health care for people with disability in the South Asian context: A review. *International Journal of Environmental Research and Public Health, 15*(11), 2366. https://doi.org/10.3390/ijerph15112366

Hendriks, A. (2007). UN convention on the rights of persons with disabilities. *European Journal of Health Law, 14*(3), 273–298. https://www.jstor.org/stable/48711822

Hornby, G. (2011). Inclusive education for children with special educational needs: A critique. *International Journal of Disability, Development and Education, 58*(3), 321–329. https://doi.org/10.1080/1034912X.2011.598678

Hulme, D. (2012). Global poverty: How global governance is failing the poor. *Routledge*. https://doi.org/10.4324/9780203844762

Ingstad, B. (2001). Disability in the developing world. In *Handbook of disability studies* (pp. 772–792). SAGE Publications, Inc. https://doi.org/10.4135/9781412976251.n35

Iravani, M., Riahi, L., Abdi, K., & Tabibi, S. J. (2021). A comparative study of the rehabilitation services systems for people with disabilities. *Archives of Rehabilitation, 21*(4), 544–563. https://doi.org/10.32598/RJ.21.4.3225.1

Jerven, M. (2013). *Poor numbers: How we are misled by African development statistics and what to do about it*. Cornell University Press.

Joint Research Centre. (2009). *Students with Disabilities, Learning difficulties and disadvantages in the Baltic States, South Eastern Europe and Malta educational policies and indicators: Educational policies and indicators* (No. 19). OECD publishing.

Kruk, H., & Waśniewska, A. (2017). Application of the Perkal method for assessing competitiveness of the countries of Central and Eastern Europe. *Oeconomia Copernicana, 8*(3), 337–352. https://doi.org/10.24136/oc.v8i3.21

Kundu, C. L. (Ed.). (2000). Status of disability in India-2000. New Delhi: Rehabilitation Council of India.

Lansdown, G. (2001). *It is our world too!: A report on the lives of disabled children*. London, UK: Disability Awareness in Action.

Lindqvist, B. (1999). Education as a fundamental right. *Education Update, 2*(4), 7.

Lishner, D. M., Richardson, M., Levine, P., & Patrick, D. (1996). Access to primary health care among persons with disabilities in rural areas: a summary of the literature. *The Journal of rural health : official journal of the American Rural Health Association and the National Rural Health Care Association, 12*(1), 45–53. https://doi.org/10.1111/j.1748-0361.1996.tb00772.x

Lyra, O., Koullapi, K., & Kalogeropoulou, E. (2023). Fears towards disability and their impact on teaching practices in inclusive classrooms: An empirical study with teachers in Greece. *Heliyon, 9*(5). https://doi.org/10.1016/j.heliyon.2023.e16332

McKinney, E. L., McKinney, V., & Swartz, L. (2021). Access to healthcare for people with disabilities in South Africa: Bad at any time, worse during COVID-19?. *South African Family Practice, 63*(3). https://doi.org/10.4102/safp.v63i1.5226

Mehrotra, N. (2011). Disability rights movements in India: Politics and practice. *Economic and Political Weekly*, 65–72.

Metts, R. L. (2000). *Disability issues, trends, and recommendations for the World Bank (full text and annexes)*. World Bank.

Mitra, S., Posarac, A., & Vick, B. C. (2011). Disability and poverty in developing countries: A snapshot from the World Health Survey. *World Bank social protection working paper*, (1109).

Mizunoya, S., & Mitra, S. (2013). Is there a disability gap in employment rates in developing countries? *World Development, 42*, 28–43. https://doi.org/10.1016/j.worlddev.2012.05.037

Moodley, J., & Ross, E. (2015). Inequities in health outcomes and access to health care in South Africa: A comparison between persons with and without disabilities. *Disability & Society, 30*(4), 630–644. https://doi.org/10.1080/09687599.2015.1034846

Murthy, G. V. S., John, N., Sagar, J., & South India Disability Evidence Study Group. (2014). Reproductive health of women with and without disabilities in South India, the SIDE study (South India Disability Evidence) study: A case control study. *BMC Women's Health, 14*, 1–7. https://doi.org/10.1186/s12905-014-0146-1

Opoku, M. P., Mprah, W. K., Dogbe, A. J., Saka, B. N., & Badu, E. (2015). Perceptions and experiences of persons with disabilities on access to education in Buea Municipality, Cameroon. *Int J Complement Alt Med, 2*(1), 207–213. https://doi.org/10.15406/ijcam.2015.02.00044

Oranga, J., & Gaungying, D. (2019). The elusiveness of inclusive education in Kenya. *Nairobi Journal of Humanities and Social Sciences, 3*(1). https://doi.org/10.58256/njhs.v3i1.806

Peprah, J. A., Avorkpo, E. A., & Kulu, E. (2023). People with disability and access to financial services: Evidence from Ghana. *Regional Science Policy & Practice, 15*(6), 1198–1216. https://doi.org/10.1111/rsp3.12643

Peters, S. (2007). Inclusion as a strategy for achieving education for all. In *The SAGE handbook of special education* (pp. 118–131). SAGE Publications Ltd. https://doi.org/10.4135/9781848607989.n10

Peters, S. J. (2003). *Inclusive education: Achieving education for all by including those with disabilities and special education needs* (pp. 1–133). World Bank.

Peters, S. J. (2004). *Inclusive education: An EFA strategy for all children*. World Bank, Human Development Network.

Peters, S., Johnstone, C., & Ferguson, P. (2005). A disability rights in education model for evaluating inclusive education. *International Journal of Inclusive Education, 9*(2), 139–160. https://doi.org/10.1080/1360311042000320464

Razzaque, M. A., & Hasan, E. (2024). Persons with disabilities in Bangladesh: Addressing gaps in data, Social protection, and Employment accessibility.

Rieser, R. (2000). History of our oppression: Why the social model in education in inclusive education. In *International Special Education Congress, Manchester, England*.

Rieser, R. (2012). *Implementing inclusive education: a Commonwealth guide to implementing Article 24 of the UN Convention on the Rights of Persons with Disabilities*. Commonwealth Secretariat. https://doi.org/10.14217/9781848591271-en

Rohwerder, B. (2015). Disability inclusion.

Sedeto, M., & Dar, M. (2019). Socioeconomic challenges of persons with disabilities: A case study of Ethiopia. *Global J Human Soc Sci, 19*(1).

Shenoy, M. (2011). *Persons with disability and the India labour market: Challenges and opportunities*. ILO, 13(1).

Suresh, V., & Dyaram, L. (2020). Workplace disability inclusion in India: Review and directions. *Management Research Review, 43*(12). https://doi.org/10.1108/MRR-11-2019-0479

Unicef. (2007). *Promoting the rights of children with disabilities United Nations International Children Emergency Fund*. Promoting the Rights of Children with Disabilities 2007.

Uriah, O. A., & Wosu, J. I. (2012). Formal education as a panacea for sustainable national development: A theoretical discussion. *International Journal of Scientific Research in Education, 5*(2), 130–137.

WHO, W. (2011). World disability report. *Malta: World Health Organisation, The World Bank*.

Wickenden, M., Thompson, S., Mader, P., Brown, S., & Rohwerder, B. (2020). Accelerating disability inclusive formal employment in Bangladesh. *Kenya, Nigeria, and Uganda: What are the vital ingredients*.

Chapter 4
Technological Innovations and Their Impact on Disability in Asian and African Continents

Abstract Telehealth and incipient technologies, particularly in Artificial Intelligence (AI), are revolutionizing accessibility and inclusion for people with disabilities (PwDs), offering transformative opportunities to overcome historical barriers. While telehealth continues to expand globally, with varying levels of integration, it remains a critical component of e-health initiatives, especially for individuals with disabilities. AI, with its capacity for natural language processing, data analytics, and machine learning, holds immense potential in reimagining the support and empowerment of disabled individuals, mainly by providing personalized, tailored solutions beyond traditional physical accommodations. This shift from conventional impairment-focused interventions to a more holistic approach considering environmental, technological, and social factors has redefined disability in a technology-driven world. In this context, information and communication technologies (ICT) and assistive technologies offer new pathways for PwDs to engage in education, employment, and social activities. However, while these innovations create new possibilities, they also introduce challenges that must be addressed to ensure equal participation and inclusion. This chapter explores the opportunities and challenges of technological advancements in fostering social development for PwDs, specifically focusing on the Asian and African continents. Examining how ICT and assistive technologies can bridge gaps and promote inclusion aims to provide insights into how technology can improve the lives of disabled individuals in these regions and contribute to an equitable, inclusive society.

Keywords Disability · Artificial intelligence · Information technology · Communication technologies · Assistive technology

4.1 Introduction

In a rapidly evolving environment filled with complex terminology, telehealth is steadily expanding in both developed and developing nations, all within the broader context of e-health. Evidence suggests that telehealth is utilized in nearly every country globally, though it remains fully integrated only in a few (Scott & Mars, 2015). This reflects a more significant trend of technological advancements reshaping societal structures, particularly concerning disabilities. Technological innovations are significantly altering both the prevalence and functional impact of child disabilities, changing the extent of social inequalities related to disability, and potentially redefining the concept of disability itself in an increasingly technology-driven world (Wise, 2012). People with disabilities are more eager than ever to engage in education, convivial activities, vocation, and ethnographic experiences. However, they face various challenges, from tangible limitations to restricted information dissemination. This is where AI plays a critical role, offering a transformative opportunity to support and foster autonomy for people with disabilities in new ways.

AI aims to enable machines, specifically computers, to mimic human thinking (Danasekaran, 2023). AI systems can process and adapt to vast amounts of data through the coalescence of computer vision, natural language processing, machine learning, and data analytics. As a result, AI leverages data to generate actionable insights and solutions that were previously unimaginable. This remarkable potential of AI can help create innovative solutions to remove barriers for entities with impairments. AI's application in the disability sector represents a fundamental transferal in how accessibility is conceptualized and implemented. While customary strategies often involve modifying the physical environment or offering limited accommodations, AI-driven solutions provide customized support beyond substantial adaptations. By embracing AI, people with disabilities are entrusted to maneuver the world in ways that meet their individual needs, overcoming historical constraints that have hindered their complete involvement (Almufareh et al., 2024).

Historically, interventions for children with disabilities were primarily aimed at addressing specific impairments or deficits. However, decades of research and advocacy have expanded this approach, incorporating a broader range of environmental and societal factors that are now seen as essential for optimizing the health, development, and social participation of children with disabilities. This more comprehensive perspective emphasizes the dynamic interaction between the physical environment, technological forces, and social factors that shape the lived experiences of disabled individuals. Today, technological innovation is not only transforming how childhood disabilities are prevented and treated, but it is also altering the scope of social disparities associated with disability. The pace and nature of these innovations are widening the impact of child disability and possibly reshaping the definition of disability itself, especially in an era where technology plays a central role in social and healthcare systems (Wise, 2012).

The guiding principle of "Disabled but not disqualified" captures the ongoing collaboration between governments, organizations, NGOs, and the private sector to help people with disabilities (PwDs) integrate into mainstream society. This partnership aims to ensure that PwDs can reach their full potential. The rise of information and communications technology (ICT) has created new possibilities for PwDs, offering them opportunities that were once out of reach. Despite the significant challenges, concerted efforts are underway to harness ICT to overcome disability-related obstacles. While the information society presents substantial opportunities for PwDs, it also introduces new barriers that must be addressed to ensure their full social inclusion (Eid, 2013).

ICT and assistive technology offer enhanced possibilities for all, but they are particularly transformative for PwDs, who depend more extensively on assistive technologies than the general population for daily activities. Modern assistive technology, designed to accommodate a wide range of abilities, enables disabled users to engage more fully in all aspects of social life than ever before. To ensure that these advancements benefit all individuals equally, providing accessibility to people with disabilities is essential to accessing the full potential of ICT and participating in an inclusive, barrier-free information society. It is crucial for enhancing social integration and creating an equitable foundation for development (Eid, 2013).

This chapter focuses on the challenges and opportunities posed by technological changes to social development, particularly in the Asian and African continents. It examines the mechanisms through which technological innovations can contribute to social development among disabled individuals, exploring how ICT and assistive technologies may help bridge existing gaps and foster greater inclusion in these regions. By considering the unique challenges disabled populations face in these continents, the chapter aims to highlight how technological advancements can be leveraged to improve the lives of disabled individuals, enabling their participation in a rapidly changing world.

4.2 Assistive Technologies: Progress and Barriers

Assistive Technologies (ATs) are tools, devices, software, or equipment designed to help individuals with disabilities perform tasks, improve their capabilities, and enhance their independence in physical and digital environments. These technologies bridge the gap between a person's abilities and the demands of their surroundings by improving communication, mobility, environmental control, and adaptive living. AI-powered assistive technologies, such as real-time object recognition for blind people, hearing aids, and customized education for people with cognitive disabilities, are helping individuals interact more effectively with their environment (Edyburn, 2000).

The rise of Machine Learning (ML) and Artificial Intelligence (AI) in Africa offers significant routes to enhance the personal welfare of PwDs by improving communication, mobility, independence, and access to digital services. However, AI systems often inherit biases from datasets that underrepresent specific communities, including PwDs. It can result in discrimination, such as PwDs being deemed unqualified by AI during recruitment processes or being unfairly affected in areas like health insurance costs and eligibility for social services (Kirongo et al., 2022).

Over 80% of PwDs live in economically disadvantaged nations, also termed as low- and middle-income countries (LMICs), where access to Assistive Technologies is limited. Research shows that many PwDs face barriers when interacting with government websites, especially in the era of e-government, leading to increased social and economic inequality. This issue became particularly evident in Kenya during the COVID-19 pandemic when government services transitioned online, excluding many disabled individuals. Additionally, AI models used in automated decision-making can misinterpret cues from people with disabilities, such as those on the autism spectrum or individuals with amputated limbs. As technology evolves in the Fourth Industrial Revolution (4IR), it is crucial to ensure that PwDs are recognized and supported by technology through accessible features and ATs to avoid further exclusion (Senjam & Manna, 2024).

Research shows that innovative digital Assistive Technologies (ATs) are being developed in Africa, though many are still in the early stages and face challenges related to sustainability. Notable advancements have been made in countries like Egypt, Ghana, Kenya, and South Africa, while most other African nations have little to no significant development or use of such technologies (Marasinghe et al., 2015). In Africa, several AI-driven assistive technologies support individuals with disabilities. The ShazaCin App in South Africa provides audio descriptions for media, aiding the blind and those with cognitive disabilities. In Ghana, Abena AI offers a hands-free offline voice assistant in Twi, and the IXAM platform helps blind students access past exam questions. Egypt's e3rafli Magnifier uses AI for object recognition to assist people who are blind. The AI4KSL project in Kenya translates spoken English to Kenyan Sign Language for deaf people, while South Africa's Senso bracelet alerts deaf users to sounds. AI also benefits those with physical disabilities. The Walk Again Project in Nigeria creates affordable 3D-printed prosthetics, integrating Brain-Machine Interface technology for mobility. Tunisia's Cure Bionics develops bionic limbs and exoskeletons using AI and 3D printing. Sierra Leone's AIMH Africa offers AI-powered mental health support for people with disabilities. Despite these innovations, many African countries lack assistive technologies, facing limited funding, policy gaps, and digital skill shortages. Most assistive tools are developed by companies outside Africa and are accessed primarily through smartphones (Josephine, 2024).

AI is progressing rapidly in Asian countries, and it is being increasingly utilized to magnify the lives of people with disabilities in innumerable modes. One key application is real-time captioning technology, which leverages AI to provide descriptors for uninterrupted audio. This technology is beneficial for individuals who are deaf in environments like classrooms, meetings, and concerts (Kawas et al., 2016; Millett, 2021). Additionally, technology-driven sign language tools can transcribe gestural language into text or convert it into oration into excerpt or discourse, facilitating communication between deaf individuals and those unfamiliar with sign language.

BCIs (brain-computer interfaces) are technologies that decode brain activity into instructions, allowing individuals to control computers or other devices. This innovation offers new possibilities for people with disabilities, particularly those with mobility limitations or severe communication disorders, to interact with the world and express themselves more easily. BCIs can help disabled individuals gain control over their surroundings and communicate with others more effectively (Cruz et al., 2021; Kinney-Lang et al., 2020).

4.2 Assistive Technologies: Progress and Barriers

AI-enhanced wheelchairs are another innovation that can navigate obstacles, avoid collisions, and even climb stairs (Rahimunnisa et al., 2020). Similarly, AI-enabled prosthetic limbs that respond to brain signals can be customized to fit the specific requirements of individual users (Elbreki et al., 2022). AI-driven eyeglasses offer features like real-time captioning translation systems for individuals with visual or hearing challenges who can instantly convert spoken words into text or vice versa, enabling smoother communication (Sneha et al., 2022). AI-driven hearing aids can be customized to reduce contextual noise and improve speech clarity. Moreover, AI-powered applications can help individuals with disabilities with errands such as reading, writing, and solving mathematical problems (Balling et al., 2021).

People with intellectual disabilities often face barriers to accessing and participating in community services due to communication challenges, cognitive impairments, sensory issues, and lack of accessibility. Therefore, AI-powered assistive technologies can lead to substantial advancements in life for individuals with disabilities by enhancing communication, mobility, emancipation, and access to essential services. While notable advancements have been made globally, especially in Africa and Asia, challenges such as biases in AI systems, limited access to resources, and a lack of infrastructure still hinder widespread adoption. It is crucial to continue developing inclusive, accessible technologies and address these barriers to ensure that PwDs are not left behind in the evolving digital landscape. With continued innovation and support, AI can bridge the gap between ability and opportunity, fostering a more inclusive society for all.

Though progress shows widespread access to AI for people with disabilities, making their lives easier, some barriers still exist to overcome. Achieving the proper harmonizing of AI-driven support with human autonomy assistance and sustaining human autonomy is a complex confrontation, requiring perpetual discussions and a focus on user-centered design principles. As AI continues to gain traction, it is critical to implement a holistic data confidentiality framework. Safeguarding sensitive personal information is paramount, ensuring it is fortified from encroachments and only used for its preordained rationale. Building trust in AI solutions demands the creation of strong data governance protocols, effective encryption, and strict adherence to regulatory standards. While AI holds a significant edge in promoting assortment and inclusion, disparities in access must be referred to proximately. Marginalized communities may encounter challenges in fully utilizing AI-driven disability aids due to disparities in digital access and limited availability of resources. The key to reducing inequalities is to guarantee affordability, fair access, and training. Overcoming these obstacles will require collaboration across various fields and sectors. Researchers, policymakers, healthcare professionals, technology innovators, and individuals with disabilities must collaborate to develop inclusive solutions, create ethical frameworks, and ensure AI technologies align with community needs and values. By embracing emerging technologies, addressing challenges head-on, and fostering innovative partnerships, we can unlock AI's full potential, creating a community where people with disabilities rise above limitations and flourish by removing impediments and advancing empowerment and inclusion (Almufareh et al.,

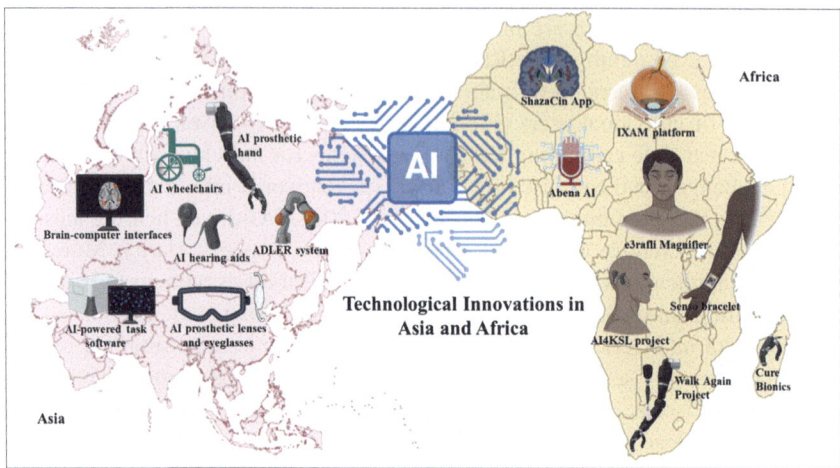

Fig. 4.1 Map illustration of technological innovations in Asia and Africa. The figure illustrates the technological advancements in assistive technology for people with disabilities across Asia and Africa. The left side represents Asian innovations, including AI-powered wheelchairs, prosthetic hands, brain-computer interfaces, AI hearing aids, and prosthetic lenses. The right side highlights African assistive technologies, such as the ShazaCin App, the IXAM platform for visual impairments, AI-powered magnifiers, smart bracelets, and advanced prosthetic limbs. The central AI symbol signifies the role of artificial intelligence in enhancing accessibility and independence for individuals with disabilities in both regions

2024). Figure 4.1 depicts the various tools and software used to enhance accessibility for people with disabilities.

4.3 AI and Robotics: Future of Accessibility

Recent advancements in robotics, particularly in assistive robotics (AR), have significantly improved the independence and quality of life of people with disabilities. These technologies have evolved from large, complex systems into more affordable, functional, and aesthetically appealing solutions, offering many benefits. AR can enhance mobility, support daily activities, assist in bowel and bladder management, relieve skin pressure, assist with vocational tasks, and facilitate better communication. These advancements enable users to re-enter the workforce, reduce caregiver burden, live independently, prevent medical complications, and improve self-image and life satisfaction. However, the appropriate prescription of robotic systems is essential for ensuring their effectiveness. When the wrong system is chosen, it can result in disuse, excessive maintenance costs, or aesthetic issues, undermining the potential benefits. Despite safety improvements, some robotic systems continue to pose injury risks to users. Furthermore, while AR systems can increase independence, they may inadvertently lead to social isolation due to reduced caregiver-interpersonal

4.3 AI and Robotics: Future of Accessibility

interaction, which poses a considerable challenge for individuals with disabilities who rely on social connections for emotional support (Costanzo et al., 2024).

Matching the right robotic device to an individual's needs presents a significant challenge. While advancements in AI are helping to create robots that assist individuals with disabilities in performing daily tasks, the process of determining the most appropriate technology is complex. These robots provide both practical support and companionship, which can be critical for helping individuals lead more independent lives. Moreover, augmented reality (AR) and virtual reality (VR) technologies are harnessed to build engaging and transformative occurrences for disabled individuals. For instance, VR can enable individuals with vision impairments to be subjected to their environment in previously impossible ways, while AR assists people with brute incapacities, allowing them to complete errands that might otherwise be insurmountable (Arvanitis et al., 2009; Tang et al., 2015).

AI-powered robotic assistants also play a critical role in supporting individuals with intellectual disabilities. These robots can assist with cooking, cleaning, and navigation tasks, enabling individuals with intellectual disabilities to perform daily activities more independently. In addition to these practical applications, these robots provide social interaction and emotional companionship, which is especially valuable for those who struggle with communication or socializing with others. These examples highlight the potential of AI to revolutionize the experiences of people with intellectual disabilities. As AI technology evolves, the range of applications supporting individuals with unique needs is anticipated to expand significantly. Autonomous systems and AI-powered robotics are also crucial in offering suppleness support to individuals with physical disabilities, enabling them to move around with greater independence (Almufareh et al., 2024).

In Asia, the application of rehabilitation robotic technologies, including therapeutic and assistive robots, has emerged as a key focus, particularly in supporting neurorehabilitation following strokes and addressing rehabilitation care gaps. These robots fall under the broader category of ATs, and notable instances include the Activities of Daily Living Exercise Robot (ADLER) system, which utilizes the Haptic-Master as a therapy robot to stipulate task-driven therapy through communal daily conducts. The BAXTER robot is also an assistive social robot designed to scrutinize and facilitate networking events (Johnson et al., 2020). Despite their potential, these robotic systems are typically found in high-income countries (HICs) due to their high cost and are often limited to hospital-affiliated outpatient clinics, large private hospitals, and other specialized settings (Mehrholz et al., 2018). Between 2003 and 2022, there has been a noticeable increase in review articles investigating the assets, value optimization, and substantiation supporting the deployment of robotic devices for rehabilitation in medical care (Veerbeek et al., 2017). Most randomized controlled trials (RCTs) have been conducted in HICs, often using exorbitant robotic rehabilitation systems. The findings from these studies show that rehabilitation robots function effectively as support tools. They work with therapists and healthcare providers to conduct quantitative assessments, deliver objective recovery data, and facilitate high-intensity, repetitive, and consistent exercise routines (Calabro et al., 2021; Stucki et al., 2007). Contrary to these positive findings, several unresolved questions remain, including identifying which patients benefit most and concerns about the optimal timing, frequency, duration, and dosage of training sessions (Stucki et al., 2007).

When considering the evidence from the International Classification of Function (ICF) perspective, rehabilitation robots have positively impacted body-level functions, such as enhancing muscle strength and motor control and improving activity levels, especially for Activities of Daily Living (ADLs). Recent advancements in wearable exoskeletons and soft robots, which can be attached to the user's body, have also improved participation. These benefits appear more pronounced in robots targeting the upper limbs than those focusing on the lower limbs. With the continued growth of the global rehabilitation robotics market, one study indicated a compound annual growth rate (CAGR) of 20.1% from 2021 to 2022, with projections suggesting the market could reach $20.8 billion by 2026. Most companies manufacturing rehabilitation robots are based in North America, Europe, and a few Asian countries, with relatively few players in Latin and South America or the Middle East and Africa. This geographical disparity in production and distribution means that access to these advanced robotic systems is unequal across regions (Islam et al., 2023; Johnson et al., 2024).

The expensive nature, intricacy, and large extent of many rehabilitation robotic systems significantly restrict their accessibility for stroke survivors in rural regions, community-based environments in high-income countries, and the vast, widely held LMICs. Consequently, the benefits of rehabilitation robotics are unevenly distributed, leaving many individuals unable to take advantage of these promising technologies. Therefore, there is an urgent need for innovative solutions to make rehabilitation robotics more accessible, especially in LMICs and rural or community-based settings within high-income countries, to bridge the existing healthcare resource gaps. These disparities in access to rehabilitation technologies are particularly noticeable in Asia and other underserved regions.

As robots become increasingly integrated into rehabilitation settings, the documented benefits of these systems must be carefully weighed against the potential risks that arise from increased human–robot interactions. Several critical concerns have emerged, including job supplanting, acquiescence, exposure, social connectedness, safety, sovereignty, empathy, legal answerability for injuries, concealment, and distributive justice. These challenges are unified, and the resolutions or guidelines proposed often vary depending on the specific type of robot and the particular medical environment in which it is used. Addressing these concerns is essential to ensuring that rehabilitation robotics continue to evolve in a way that benefits all individuals, regardless of their geographical location or socioeconomic status. As AI and robotics continue to advance, these technologies will convalesce the existences of people with infirmities dramatically, but efforts must be made to make these solutions more inclusive and accessible worldwide (Johnson & Mendonca, 2023).

Therefore, when comparing Asia and Africa regarding the adoption and use of rehabilitation robotics, several key differences arise, primarily due to variations in socioeconomic conditions, infrastructure, and access to technology. In Asia, countries like Japan, South Korea, and China have made significant progress in developing and deploying rehabilitation robotics, driven by substantial investments in research and innovation. These technologies are most commonly found in urban areas and high-income settings, although efforts are underway to extend their reach to rural communities. On the other hand, Africa faces more substantial obstacles in the widespread adoption of rehabilitation robotics, mainly due to financial constraints, inadequate infrastructure, and limited technological advancements in the field. The rehabilitation robotics market in Africa remains underdeveloped, and the high costs of these systems present significant barriers to access, particularly in low-income and rural areas. While both regions struggle with unequal access to advanced rehabilitation technologies, Asia's more advanced technological infrastructure and significant research investments offer a more promising outlook for expanding these solutions. At the same time, Africa needs targeted strategies to address the technological divide and improve healthcare access across the continent. Table 4.1 presents various software developments to enhance accessibility for people with disabilities in public spaces.

4.4 The Role of Telemedicine and Digital Health

Access to healthcare is a critical factor influencing health outcomes. The COVID-19 pandemic has accelerated the shift toward virtual telemedicine, replacing customary in-person appointments due to social distancing requirements. While telemedicine has improved access and reduced barriers for many, individuals with disabilities still face significant challenges, and new obstacles have emerged during the pandemic, some of which may persist for the foreseeable future. People with disabilities constitute an economically vulnerable population encountering distinct social and environmental challenges. They experience healthcare inconsistencies that affect access, deteriorate their health, and ultimately result in poorer health outcomes compared to individuals without disabilities (Smith, 2019). In the U.S., 61 million adults live with a disability. Those with disabilities are generally older, have lower incomes, and experience higher rates of heart disease, diabetes, obesity, and smoking (Mack, 2023). They are also less likely to have a consistent healthcare provider, struggle more with affording healthcare, and are more likely to have unmet healthcare needs. Furthermore, there is a more significant proportion of individuals with disabilities in rural areas compared to urban areas (Centers for Disease Control and Prevention, 2016).

Before the pandemic, telemedicine served as a substitute for in-person healthcare. If a person with a disability encountered difficulties accessing or communicating with healthcare providers through telemedicine, they could still opt for in-person care. However, these challenges must be addressed, with telemedicine now emerging as the primary and often sole healthcare access method. Implementing new safeguards and measures to promote healthcare equity through telemedicine is essential. In the post-COVID-19 era, telemedicine should no longer be viewed as a mere supplement to in-person visits but as a viable alternative, given its anticipated continued use even as traditional healthcare appointments return. This transition requires addressing

Table 4.1 Various software developments designed to enhance accessibility for people with disabilities in public spaces

Category	Tool name	Application	Challenges	Focussed areas
Assistive Technology	ShazaCin	Provides audio descriptions for media to assist people who are blind and those with cognitive disabilities	Limited access to smartphones and the Internet for many PwDs; technology underdevelopment in other regions	South Africa
Assistive Technology	Abena AI	Offers a hands-free, offline voice assistant in Twi to assist individuals with disabilities	Limited availability of offline solutions; reliance on smartphones	Ghana
Assistive Technology	Walk Again Project	3D-printed prosthetics with Brain-Machine Interface technology to assist mobility	High cost of technology; limited access to 3D printing resources in rural areas	Nigeria
Assistive Technology	Senso Bracelet	Alerts deaf users to sounds, such as alarms, and helps them navigate environments	Lack of widespread access to the device; costs may limit adoption in low-income settings	South Africa
Assistive Technology	e3rafli Magnifier	Uses AI for object recognition to assist people who are blind in identifying objects	Limited smartphone access; underdeveloped infrastructure for support services	Egypt
Assistive Technology	AI4KSL	Translates spoken English into Kenyan Sign Language for the deaf	Limited Internet access in rural areas; need for more language support beyond Kenyan Sign Language	Kenya
Assistive Technology	IXAM Platform	Helps blind students access past exam questions via AI-powered technology	Accessibility limitations for rural students: smartphone dependency	Ghana

(continued)

4.4 The Role of Telemedicine and Digital Health

Table 4.1 (continued)

Category	Tool name	Application	Challenges	Focussed areas
Assistive Technology	AI-driven Prosthetics	AI-powered prosthetic limbs that respond to brain signals for movement and adjustment	High cost and accessibility issues in LMICs; limited availability in rural areas	Global
Assistive Technology	AI-powered Hearing Aids	Customizes hearing aids to reduce contextual noise and enhance speech clarity	High costs; availability limited in rural areas and economically disadvantaged regions	Global
Assistive Technology	Brain-Computer Interfaces (BCI)	Allows individuals with severe disabilities to control devices via brain activity	High cost; complex technology requires specific infrastructure and training	Global
Rehabilitation Robotics	Rehabilitation Robots (e.g., ADLER System, HapticMaster)	Assists in neurorehabilitation and daily living exercises, improving motor control and strength	High cost; limited availability in rural or low-income areas; accessibility issues for stroke patients	Asia (Japan, South Korea, China)
Rehabilitation Robotics	BAXTER Robot	Assistive social robot for networking events helps disabled individuals with social interactions	High cost and infrastructure limitations, primarily found in specialized environments	Asia (Japan, South Korea, China)
Rehabilitation Robotics	Soft Exoskeletons	Wearable robots that assist with mobility and rehabilitation	High production costs; lack of widespread availability in LMICs; dependency on specialized care	Global
Assistive Technology	Cure Bionics	Develops bionic limbs using AI and 3D printing to assist those with limb amputations	High cost; limited access to 3D printing and technical expertise in low-income areas	Tunisia

(continued)

Table 4.1 (continued)

Category	Tool name	Application	Challenges	Focussed areas
Assistive Technology	AIMH Africa	Provides AI-powered mental health support for individuals with disabilities	Access to technology and data privacy concerns; limited availability in rural areas	Sierra Leone
AI & Robotics	AI-Powered Captioning	Provides real-time captioning for individuals who are deaf or hard of hearing in various environments	Limited access in rural areas; technology may misinterpret non-standard speech or accents	Global
AI & Robotics	AI-powered Translation Systems	Translates spoken words into text or vice versa for individuals with hearing or visual impairments	Misinterpretation of speech or gestures; limited technology in rural settings	Global
AI & Robotics	VR for Vision Impairments	Provides an immersive experience for visually impaired individuals to interact with their environment	Expensive equipment; accessibility in low-income and rural areas	Global

several related issues (Gilbert et al., 2020). Historically, the challenges related to healthcare access for people with disabilities focused on in-person visits, particularly considering (a) Tangible admittance to healthcare facilities, (b) Equipment used for interactions between patients and providers, and (c) Communication and educational tools for patients. These topics need to be revisited at this juncture, considering the central role of telemedicine in healthcare access, which is likely to remain a critical component even beyond the pandemic.

Telemedicine offers several potential benefits for people with disabilities, including lower healthcare costs, reduced transportation expenses, improved communication for pharmaceutical synchronization, diminished revelation to contagious sicknesses (particularly in times of a pandemic), and a reduced necessity for remunerated respective aid (Agha et al., 2002). However, given the contemporary focus on telemedicine, it is an opportune time to methodically evaluate its provisions, perils, and potential for enhancing medical encounters for those with disabilities.

Telemedicine programs are not new in healthcare organizations across Sub-Saharan Africa (SSA). These programs have significantly strengthened healthcare systems, promoted care recipients and professional health education, and supported disease surveillance and prevention in the region (Dodoo et al., 2021). Telemedicine

4.4 The Role of Telemedicine and Digital Health

systems were wildly successful in combating the Ebola virus in some areas of Africa (Ohannessian, 2015). Recent research suggests a renewed emphasis on the adoption of telemedicine in Sub-Saharan Africa (SSA), particularly as an alternative healthcare delivery model during the COVID-19 pandemic (Behar et al., 2020; Webster, 2020). This shift has been facilitated by the widespread use of mobile telecommunications across SSA nations. Holst et al., (2020) highlighted that telemedicine could revolutionize healthcare delivery in SSA. Their study revealed that 41 countries in the region have established national digital health strategies and frameworks (NDHSA), and mobile phone connections, which totaled 816 million in 2019, are projected to reach 1.05 billion by 2025 (Adepoju, 2020), facilitating more significant use of telemedicine applications.

However, the authors pointed out a significant gap in research regarding the progress of telemedicine, specifically the lack of baseline studies to assess users' gratification with telemedicine amenities. Adebayo et al., (2021) focused their research on teleneurology and the readiness of infrastructure in SSA, which limits the scope of understanding regarding telemedicine implementation across the region. Furthermore, prior literature has often examined telemedicine adoption fragmentally, focusing on specific services or countries, leading to inconsistent findings across SSA. This gap provides a prospect for reviewing the overall enhancement of telemedicine programs and the disputes involved in their implementation in SSA.

The findings from such a review could provide timely guidance for policymakers on the current state of telemedicine implementation and highlight opportunities for regional collaboration. It could also outline the assorted approaches to telemedicine rollout, potentially helping to address common issues or redundancies observed in telemedicine systems in some SSA countries, such as South Africa (Dodoo et al., 2022).

The Asian continent is well known for telemedicine, where different types of telemedicine are carried out to monitor patients. Teleconsultation refers to consultations between patients and remote physicians, and Teletherapy involves patients receiving instructions or home exercises that are demonstrated or supervised by therapists remotely. One local study examined multi-disciplinary telerehabilitation sessions, where occupational therapists, physical therapists, psychologists, physiatrists, and rehabilitation nurses collaborated in a remote community. Another study focused on teletherapy, and two studies focused on psychologists, while the others involved speech-language pathologists. Telementoring consists of a situation where a remote expert guides a healthcare provider or physician who is physically with the patient in a rural area. On the other hand, telemonitoring uses devices or online applications to allow for the remote and asynchronous transmission of health data or patient reminders (Leochico et al., 2020).

In the local studies, the paramount generic modus of implementing telerehabilitation (such as telementoring, teletherapy, teleconsultation, and telemonitoring) included mobile text messaging (SMS) (Gavino et al., 2008; Macrohon & Cristobal, 2011, 2013; Sahu et al., 2014), followed by video calls and instantaneous messaging through popular social media platforms like Viber™ (Leochico & Valera, 2020), Skype™ (Leochico & Mojica, 2017), and FaceTime™ (Villafania, 2018). Two studies coalesced web-based services (like Moodle™) with SMS for teleconsultations (Macrohon & Cristobal, 2011, 2013). In general, patients and rural physicians reported positive experiences with telerehabilitation. Concerns are primarily centered around Internet speed and data privacy challenges. Additional research has explored areas related to the acceptance of telerehabilitation and the governance of telehealth (Brieux et al., 2017; Fernandez-Marcelo et al., 2012; Marcelo, 2010; Marcelo et al., 2011; Wickramasinghe, 2008), national policies or programs (Ho et al., 2016; Marcelo et al., 2015; Patdu & Tenorio, 2016), legal concerns, as well as issues surrounding data privacy and security (Bitsch et al., 2015; Caranguian et al., 2012; Patdu & Tenorio, 2016) and ethical dilemmas (Patdu & Tenorio, 2016; Umali et al., 2016).

A number of the researchers involved in these studies were associated with the National Telehealth Center at the National Institutes of Health, University of the Philippines, Manila. According to Patdu and Tenorio (2016), although no specific telehealth legislation has been enacted in the Philippines, there have been preliminary efforts to promote telehealth by tackling ethical, legal, financial, and administrative issues. Research forums, stakeholder meetings, campaigns, and conferences organized by Fernandez-Marcelo et al. in 2012 played a key role in increasing local awareness of telehealth. The National Telehealth Service Program of the Department of Health marked a significant benchmark in raising telehealth awareness, especially in rural areas, as evidenced by studies conducted by Macrohon and Cristobal (2011) and Gavino et al., (2008). Additionally, local studies by Leochico and Mojica (2017) and Leochico and Valera (2020) contributed to raising awareness of telerehabilitation in particular. Two unpublished reviews indicated favorable attitudes toward telerehabilitation, though they highlighted limited experience among allied rehabilitation professionals in developing nations. However, no published studies specifically examined the attitudes, knowledge, and perceptions of healthcare professionals in the Philippines regarding telerehabilitation. Mandirola-Brieux et al., (2017) pointed out that cultural factors could affect the concurrence of e-health programs. According to a systematic review of telehealth in African and Asian regions, mobile text messaging emerged as the most widely embraced modus, particularly by patients with disabilities.

While telemedicine presents many potential benefits, there are challenges in its application for individuals with intellectual and developmental disabilities (IDD). For instance, people with disabilities are 20% less likely to own computers, tablets, or smartphones than those without disabilities, creating obstacles to accessing telehealth services (Perrin & Atske, 2021). Our research shows a higher adoption rate of telemedicine among individuals with IDD compared to the general population, indicating that, with the proper support, people with IDD can effectively use modern technology. However, using digital technology also presents unique risks for individuals with IDD, which may be more pronounced than those faced by the general population. One issue is how specific applications manage sensitive personal data, potentially using it for commercial purposes. People with intellectual disabilities might struggle to fully comprehend the privacy policies of these apps, making them more vulnerable to exploitation (Hatef et al., 2022).

Furthermore, communication challenges experienced by individuals with IDD (Shnamugam et al., 2014) could result in diagnostic mistakes during telemedicine consultations. Telemedicine services provided by non-routine care providers have been associated with a greater need for in-person follow-ups, raising concerns about patient safety. However, these risks can be mitigated when telehealth is offered by clinicians who are part of the patient's established care team, as they can access medical records, conduct necessary tests, offer follow-up care, and make referrals to specialists. Incorporating telemedicine as a supplementary service alongside in-person care can improve healthcare delivery for individuals with IDD (Hatef et al., 2022).

4.5 Overcoming the Digital Divide: Equitable Access to Innovations

The Advisory Commission on Consumer Protection and Quality in the Health Care Industry has identified various factors that increase an individual's susceptibility to healthcare quality issues. These factors include age, financial situation, health, geographic location, functional or communication ability, progressive repute, ethnicity, race, and gender. The Commission also highlighted that the changing healthcare system, especially the shrinking safety net, can interact with these personal factors, making individuals even more vulnerable to healthcare quality challenges (President's Advisory Commission on Consumer Protection & Quality in the Health Care Industry, 1998). Vulnerable populations are often diverse in various ways. While diversity is usually defined by social and demographic factors such as age, gender, race, ethnicity, and socioeconomic status, the Committee on Communication for Behavior Change in the 21st Century has pointed out the limitations of these definitions. They argue that communication interventions, especially those involving technology, should also consider other essential aspects of diversity. These include cultural processes, the life experiences of the communities and individuals being served, the sociocultural context, economic conditions, community resources, and shared beliefs, norms, and practices related to specific health issues (Institute of Medicine, 2002).

"Underserved population" is often used interchangeably with "vulnerable population," but they represent distinct concepts. Underserved populations specifically refer to those who receive insufficient healthcare services to address their health needs. The Health Resources and Services Administration defines medically underserved populations as groups facing economic, cultural, or linguistic barriers that hinder their access to primary medical care services (Shin et al., 2008). While there is a significant intersection between susceptible and neglected populations, it is essential to note that an individual can be vulnerable without being underserved. For example, a premature African-American infant in a neonatal intensive care unit receiving excellent care may be considered vulnerable but not underserved. However, individuals who are both deprived and fragile are at a higher risk of negative healthiness sequels and need more extensive health statistics support.

Current assessments strongly indicate that healthcare incongruences persist in the United States, particularly among underprivileged groups. These groups typically include ethnic minorities, people with low incomes, low educational or literacy levels, those living in rural areas, older people, and individuals with disabilities (Nelson, 2002; US Department of Health & Human Services, 2020). Within this context, the AMIA Spring Congress concentrated on vulnerable populations exhibiting considerable diversity and facing insufficient healthcare services. The Congress assumed that these populations, who often experience disparities in health outcomes, could benefit from greater access to pertinent health statistics and resources. The challenge of addressing these disparities has increasingly focused on how information technology, including the Internet, can be leveraged to bridge gaps in health service delivery, especially for underserved and vulnerable populations.

This challenge has led to the introduction of the term "Digital Divide," which refers to unequal availability of IT, especially the Internet, for specific groups such as ethnic and racial minorities, people with disabilities, rural communities, and those with lower socioeconomic status. A report called "Falling Through the Net: Toward Digital Inclusion" emphasized that Hispanic and Black populations are significantly less likely than the national average to own computers, have Internet access, or use the Internet at home (National Telecommunications & Information Administration, 2000). However, more recent data from the Pew Internet and American Life Project indicate a change in this pattern. While 75% of Hispanics use computers (surpassing the 73% of whites and 62% of blacks), Hispanics still lag slightly behind whites in Internet usage (63% vs. 64%). The data further shows that while Internet access has risen across all income brackets, it remains disproportionately higher among wealthier households. For instance, 89% of homes with incomes over $75,000 have Internet access, compared to just 55% of those under $30,000. Furthermore, Internet usage is higher in urban areas (65%) compared to rural areas (48%) (Horrigan, 2004). The number of seniors using the Internet has also increased, with 22% now online, and of these "connected" seniors, 66% use the Internet to search for health-related information (Fox, 2004).

As Internet access has expanded, new aspects of the digital divide have surfaced, including health literacy, computer literacy, and the gap between available and desired e-health services. According to The Children's Partnership, at least 50 million Americans (or 20% of the population) encounter obstacles that prevent them from fully utilizing the Internet. These barriers include a dearth of local information (21 million), literacy challenges (44 million), language barriers (32 million), and a paucity of cultural diversity in content (26 million) (Lazarus & Mora, 2000). The Institute of Medicine (IOM) Committee on Health Literacy further emphasized that health literacy is shaped by educational, cultural, social, and health service factors, meaning it is not merely an individual trait (Kindig et al., 2004). It is particularly relevant to vulnerable populations, who often struggle with accessing and interpreting health information due to these compounding factors.

Multiple government agencies and collaborative partnerships are working to close the healthcare information and communication access gap. Efforts are being made at the state, regional, national, and medical center levels to evaluate the effect of information technology on health outcomes. Despite these initiatives, many underserved populations still face obstacles in accessing or effectively using health information. However, digital access has increased across most demographic groups, and a digital divide persists, particularly affecting the most vulnerable populations. This ongoing issue was a significant focus of the Spring Congress, which addressed the need for more inclusive approaches to healthcare delivery and information access for underserved and vulnerable groups (Chang et al., 2004).

A study in Africa further explores the digital divide issue in an educational context. The study assessed postgraduate students' information literacy (IL) skills, awareness of IL classes, and the perceived need for such training at the University of the Western Cape (UWC). The findings revealed that many postgraduate students lacked confidence in their IL skills and struggled to use electronic tools. This study highlights UWC Library's efforts to bridge the digital divide by addressing postgraduate students' lack of awareness and skills related to electronic resources, such as e-books and online tools. The library actively integrates IL into the broader curriculum and collaborates with various networks to promote lifelong learning. Key initiatives such as training in reference management systems, the introduction of the Ekamva LMS, device loan programs, and the Digital Academic Literacy (DAL) course support students' access to ICT tools and resources. Despite challenges, such as limited access to QR code services and other technological issues, UWC's ongoing projects aim to enhance digital literacy and ensure equitable access to education for all students, particularly those from historically disadvantaged backgrounds (Nyahodza & Higgs, 2017).

Therefore, the digital divide remains a critical issue affecting healthcare and education, particularly for vulnerable and underserved populations. While there have been significant advancements in access to technology, ongoing efforts are needed to bridge gaps in digital literacy, health literacy, and the availability of digital resources. The work done by UWC Library, as well as similar initiatives globally, underscores the importance of providing both the tools and the training necessary to empower individuals, especially from marginalized communities, to benefit fully from the opportunities offered by digital technologies.

4.6 Conclusion

The advancement of technology, particularly that of AI and ICT, presents unprecedented opportunities for improving the quality of life of people with disabilities in Asia and Africa. Assistive technologies, AI-powered robotics, and telemedicine promise greater inclusion, independence, and improved health outcomes. However, realizing this potential requires overcoming substantial challenges. The digital divide, characterized by unequal access to technology and digital literacy, remains a significant barrier. Biases embedded within AI systems can lead to discrimination and further marginalization.

Furthermore, limited resources and infrastructure, particularly in many parts of Africa, hinder the widespread adoption of these life-changing technologies. The high cost of advanced rehabilitation robotics, for example, restricts access primarily to high-income countries and settings. A holistic approach is needed to address these challenges. Governments must invest in policies that promote inclusivity and accessibility, infrastructure development, and digital literacy programs. Researchers and technology developers must prioritize inclusive design principles, ensuring that AI systems are free from bias and cater to the diverse needs of PwDs. International collaborations are essential to sharing knowledge, resources, and best practices. Finally, empowering PwDs through active participation in designing and implementing these technologies is imperative to confirm their practicality and efficiency. Only through sustained effort and collaborative action can we harness the transformative power of technology to create a truly inclusive society where PwDs can thrive and reach their full potential.

References

Adebayo, P. B., Oluwole, O. J., & Taiwo, F. T. (2021). COVID-19 and teleneurology in Sub-Saharan Africa: Leveraging the current exigency. *Frontiers in Public Health, 8*, Article 574505. https://doi.org/10.3389/fpubh.2020.574505

Adepoju, P. (2020). Africa turns to telemedicine to close mental health gap. *The Lancet Digital Health, 2*(11), e571–e572. https://doi.org/10.1016/S2589-7500(20)30252-1

Agha, Z., Schapira, R. M., & Maker, A. H. (2002). Cost effectiveness of telemedicine for the delivery of outpatient pulmonary care to a rural population. *Telemedicine Journal and e-Health, 8*(3), 281–291. https://doi.org/10.1089/15305620260353171

Almufareh, M. F., Kausar, S., Humayun, M., & Tehsin, S. (2024). A conceptual model for inclusive technology: Advancing disability inclusion through artificial intelligence. *Journal of Disability Research, 3*(1), 20230060. https://doi.org/10.57197/JDR-2023-0060

Arvanitis, T. N., Petrou, A., Knight, J. F., Savas, S., Sotiriou, S., Gargalakos, M., & Gialouri, E. (2009). Human factors and qualitative pedagogical evaluation of a mobile augmented reality system for science education used by learners with physical disabilities. *Personal and Ubiquitous Computing, 13*, 243–250. https://doi.org/10.1007/s00779-007-0187-7

Balling, L. W., Mølgaard, L. L., Townend, O., & Nielsen, J. B. B. (2021, August). The collaboration between hearing aid users and artificial intelligence to optimize sound. *Seminars in Hearing, 42*(3), 282–294. https://doi.org/10.1055/s-0041-1735135

Behar, J. A., Liu, C., Kotzen, K., Tsutsui, K., Corino, V. D., Singh, J., Pimentel, M. A. F., Warrick, P., Zaunseder, S., Andreotti, F., Sebag, D., Kopanitsa, G., McSharry, P. E., Karlen, W., Karmakar, C., & Clifford, G. D. (2020). Remote health monitoring and diagnosis in the time of COVID-19. *arXiv preprint* arXiv:2005.08537. https://doi.org/10.1088/1361-6579/abba0a

Bitsch, J. Á., Ramos, R., Ix, T., Ferrer-Cheng, P. G., & Wehrle, K. (2015). Psychologist in a pocket: Towards depression screening on mobile phones. In *pHealth 2015* (pp. 153–159). IOS Press. https://doi.org/10.3233/978-1-61499-516-6-153

Calabro, R. S., Sorrentino, G., Cassio, A., Mazzoli, D., Andrenelli, E., Bizzarini, E., & Bonaiuti, D. (2021). Robotic-assisted gait rehabilitation following stroke: a systematic review of current guidelines and practical clinical recommendations. *European Journal of Physical and Rehabilitation Medicine, 57*(3), 460–471. https://doi.org/10.23736/s1973-9087.21.06887-8

Caranguian, L. P. R., Pancho-Festin, S., & Sison, L. G. (2012, August). Device interoperability and authentication for telemedical appliance based on the ISO/IEEE 11073 personal health device (PHD) standards. In *2012 Annual International Conference of the IEEE Engineering in Medicine and Biology Society* (pp. 1270–1273). IEEE. https://doi.org/10.1109/embc.2012.6346169

Centers for Disease Control and Prevention. (2016). Prevalence of disability and disability types by urban-rural county classification—United States. Accessed May 18, 2020. https://www.cdc.gov/ncbddd/disabilityandhealth/features/disabilityprevalence-rural-urban.html. Accessed November 18, 2019

Chang, B. L., Bakken, S., Brown, S. S., Houston, T. K., Kreps, G. L., Kukafka, R., & Stavri, P. Z. (2004). Bridging the digital divide: Reaching vulnerable populations. *Journal of the American Medical Informatics Association, 11*(6), 448–457. https://doi.org/10.1197/jamia.m1535

Costanzo, M., Smeriglio, R., & Di Nuovo, S. (2024). New technologies and assistive robotics for elderly: A review on psychological variables. *Archives of Gerontology and Geriatrics plus, 100056*,. https://doi.org/10.1016/j.aggp.2024.100056

Cruz, A., Pires, G., Lopes, A., Carona, C., & Nunes, U. J. (2021). A self-paced BCI with a collaborative controller for highly reliable wheelchair driving: Experimental tests with physically disabled individuals. *IEEE Transactions on Human-Machine Systems, 51*(2), 109–119. https://doi.org/10.1109/THMS.2020.3047597

Danasekaran, R. (2023). The emergence of artificial intelligence in healthcare: Current trends and future directions. *Soc Determinants Health, 9*(1):1–2. https://doi.org/10.22037/sdh.v9i1.41516

Dodoo, J. E., Al-Samarraie, H., & Alsswey, A. (2022). The development of telemedicine programs in Sub-Saharan Africa: Progress and associated challenges. *Health and Technology, 12*(1), 33–46. https://doi.org/10.1007/s12553-021-00626-7

Dodoo, J. E., Al-Samarraie, H., & Alzahrani, A. I. (2021). Telemedicine use in Sub-Saharan Africa: Barriers and policy recommendations for Covid-19 and beyond. *International Journal of Medical Informatics, 151*, Article 104467. https://doi.org/10.1016/j.ijmedinf.2021.104467

Edyburn, D. L. (2000). Assistive technology and students with mild disabilities. *Focus on Exceptional Children, 32*(9). https://doi.org/10.17161/foec.v32i9.6776

Eid, N. (2013). Innovation and technology for persons with disabilities. *KN4DC project, UN-ESCWA, Chairman of Studies Center for Handicapped Research and Consultant in ICT for inclusion and development PwDs.*

Elbreki, A. M., Ramdan, S., Mohamed, F., Alshari, K., Rajab, Z., & Elhub, B. (2022, July). Practical design of an upper prosthetic limb using three dimensional printer with an artificial intelligence based controller. In *2022 International Conference on Engineering & MIS (ICEMIS)* (pp. 1–6). IEEE. https://doi.org/10.1109/ICEMIS56295.2022.9914291

Fernandez-Marcelo, P. G., Ho, B. L., Faustorilla, J. F., Jr., Evangelista, A. L., Pedrena, M., & Marcelo, A. (2012). Emerging eHealth directions in the Philippines. *Yearbook of Medical Informatics, 21*(01), 144–152. https://doi.org/10.1055/s-0038-1639446

Fox, S. (2004). Older Americans and the Internet: Adapting Government Websites for an Older Audience.

Gavino, A. I., Tolentino, P. A., Bernal, A. B., Fontelo, P., & Marcelo, A. B. (2008, November). Telemedicine via Short Messaging System (SMS) in rural Philippines. In *AMIA Annual Symposium Proceedings. AMIA Symposium* (pp. 952–952).

Gilbert, A. W., Billany, J. C., Adam, R., Martin, L., Tobin, R., Bagdai, S., & Bateson, J. (2020). Rapid implementation of virtual clinics due to COVID-19: Report and early evaluation of a quality improvement initiative. *BMJ Open Quality, 9*(2), Article e000985. https://doi.org/10.1136/bmjoq-2020-000985

Hatef, E., Lans, D., Bandeian, S., Lasser, E. C., Goldsack, J., & Weiner, J. P. (2022). Outcomes of in-person and telehealth ambulatory encounters during COVID-19 within a large commercially insured cohort. *JAMA Network Open, 5*(4), e228954–e228954. https://doi.org/10.1001/jamane tworkopen.2022.8954

Ho, K., Al-Shorjabji, N., Brown, E., Zelmer, J., Gabor, N., Maeder, A., Marcelo, A., & Doyle, T. (2016). Applying the resilient health system framework for universal health coverage. In *The promise of new technologies in an age of new health challenges* (pp. 54–62). IOS Press. https://doi.org/10.3233/978-1-61499-712-2-54

Holst, C., Sukums, F., Radovanovic, D., Ngowi, B., Noll, J., & Winkler, A. S. (2020). Sub-Saharan Africa—The new breeding ground for global digital health. *The Lancet Digital Health, 2*(4), e160–e162. https://doi.org/10.1016/S2589-7500(20)30027-3

Horrigan, J. B. (2004). PEW Internet data project memo: Home broadband adoption has increased 60% in the past year and use of DSL lines is surging.

Institute of Medicine. (2002). Committee on communication for behavior change in the 21st Century: Improving the health of diverse populations. *Speaking of health: Assessing health communication strategies for diverse populations.* https://doi.org/10.17226/10018

Islam, M. J. A., Mahmud, I., Islam, A., Sobhani, F. A., Hassan, M. S., & Ahsan, A. (2023). Escaping the middle-income trap: A study on a developing economy. *Cogent Social Sciences, 9*(2), 2286035. https://doi.org/10.1080/23311886.2023.2286035

Johnson, M. J., & Mendonca, R. J. (Eds.). (2023). *Rehabilitation Robots for neurorehabilitation in high-, low-, and middle-income countries: Current practice, barriers, and future directions.* Academic Press.

Johnson, M. J., Bui, K., & Rahimi, N. (2020). Medical and assistive robotics in global health. *Handbook of Global Health, 1–46,.* https://doi.org/10.1007/978-3-030-45009-0_76

Johnson, M. J., Keyvanian, S., & Mendonca, R. J. (2024). Toward inclusive rehabilitation robots. In *Rehabilitation robots for neurorehabilitation in high-, low-, and middle-income countries* (pp. 471–498). Academic Press.

Josephine, K. (2024). AI assistive technologies (Ats) for persons with disabilities (Pwds) in Africa. *Centre for Intellectual Property and Information Technology Law.* https://doi.org/10.1007/978-3-031-47997-7_3

Kawas, S., Karalis, G., Wen, T., & Ladner, R. E. (2016, October). Improving real-time captioning experiences for deaf and hard of hearing students. In *Proceedings of the 18th International ACM SIGACCESS Conference on Computers and Accessibility* (pp. 15–23). https://doi.org/10.1145/2982142.2982164

Kindig, D. A., Panzer, A. M., & Nielsen-Bohlman, L. (Eds.). (2004). Health literacy: A prescription to end confusion.

Kinney-Lang, E., Kelly, D., Floreani, E. D., Jadavji, Z., Rowley, D., Zewdie, E. T., & Kirton, A. (2020). Advancing brain-computer interface applications for severely disabled children through a multidisciplinary national network: Summary of the inaugural pediatric BCI Canada meeting. *Frontiers in Human Neuroscience, 14*, Article 593883. https://doi.org/10.3389/fnhum.2020.593883

Kirongo, A. C., Huka, G., Bundi, D., Kitaria, D., & Muchiri, G. (2022). Implementation of AI-based assistive technologies for learners with physical disabilities in areas of innovation and special schools: a practical design thinking approach. *African Journal of Science, Technology and Social Sciences, 1*(2), 73–76. https://doi.org/10.58506/ajstss.v1i2.124

Lazarus, W., & Mora, F. (2000). Online content for low-income and underserved Americans: The digital divide's New Frontier. A strategic audit of activities and opportunities.

Leochico, C. F. D., & Valera, M. J. S. (2020). Follow-up consultations through telerehabilitation for wheelchair recipients with paraplegia in a developing country: A case report. *Spinal Cord Series and Cases, 6*(1), 58. https://doi.org/10.1038/s41394-020-0310-9

Leochico, C. F. D., Espiritu, A. I., Ignacio, S. D., & Mojica, J. A. P. (2020). Challenges to the emergence of telerehabilitation in a developing country: A systematic review. *Frontiers in Neurology, 11*, 1007. https://doi.org/10.3389/fneur.2020.01007

Leochico, C. F., & Mojica, J. A. (2017). Telerehabilitation as a teaching-learning tool for medical interns. *PARM Proceedings, 9*(1), 39–43. https://doi.org/10.1097/PHM.0000000000001755

References

Mack, M. (2023). *Prevalence of loneliness among divorced adults*. California State University.

Macrohon, B. C., & Cristobal, F. L. (2011). Rural healthcare delivery using a phone patch service in the teleconsultation program of the Ateneo de Zamboanga University School of Medicine in Western Mindanao, Philippines. *Rural and Remote Health, 11*(2), 279–280. https://doi.org/10.22605/RRH1740

Macrohon, B. C., & Cristobal, F. L. (2013). The effect on patient and health provider satisfaction regarding health care delivery using the teleconsultation program of the Ateneo de Zamboanga University-School of Medicine (ADZU-SOM) in rural Western Mindanao. *Acta Medica Philippina, 47*(4), 18–22.

Mandirola Brieux, H. F., Benitez, S., Otero, C., Luna, D., Masud, J. H. B., Marcelo, A., & Gonzalez Bernaldo de Quirós, F. (2017). Cultural problems associated with the implementation of eHealth. In *MEDINFO 2017: Precision healthcare through informatics* (pp. 1213–1213). IOS Press.

Marasinghe, K. M., Lapitan, J. M., & Ross, A. (2015). Assistive technologies for ageing populations in six low-income and middle-income countries: A systematic review. *BMJ Innovations, 1*(4). https://doi.org/10.1136/bmjinnov-2015-000065

Marcelo, A. B. (2010). Health information systems: A survey of frameworks for developing countries. *Yearbook of Medical Informatics, 19*(01), 25–29. https://doi.org/10.1055/s-0038-1638684

Marcelo, A., Adejumo, A., & Luna, D. (2011). Health informatics for development: A threepronged strategy of partnerships, standards, and mobile Health. *Yearbook of Medical Informatics, 20*(01), 96–101. https://doi.org/10.1055/s-0038-1638745

Marcelo, A., Ganesh, J., Mohan, J., Kadam, D. B., Ratta, B. S., Kulatunga, G., & Marcelo, P. (2015). Governance and management of national telehealth programs in Asia. In *Global Telehealth 2015: Integrating Technology and Information for Better Healthcare* (pp. 95–101). IOS Press. https://doi.org/10.3233/978-1-61499-505-0-95

Mehrholz, J., Pohl, M., Platz, T., Kugler, J., & Elsner, B. (2018). Electromechanical and robot-assisted arm training for improving activities of daily living, arm function, and arm muscle strength after stroke. *Cochrane Database of Systematic Reviews, 9*. https://doi.org/10.1002/14651858.cd006876.pub5

Millett, P. (2021). Accuracy of speech-to-text captioning for students who are deaf or hard of hearing. *Journal of Educational, Pediatric & (Re) Habilitative Audiology, 25*.

Nelson, A. (2002). Unequal treatment: Confronting racial and ethnic disparities in health care. *Journal of the National Medical Association, 94*(8), 666.

Nyahodza, L., & Higgs, R. (2017). Towards bridging the digital divide in post-apartheid South Africa: A case of a historically disadvantaged university in Cape Town. *South African Journal of Libraries and Information Science, 83*(1), 39–48. https://doi.org/10.7553/83-1-1645

Ohannessian, R. (2015). Telemedicine: Potential applications in epidemic situations. *European Research in Telemedicine/la Recherche Européenne En Télémédecine, 4*(3), 95–98. https://doi.org/10.1016/j.eurtel.2015.08.002

Patdu, I. D., & Tenorio, A. S. (2016). Establishing the legal framework of telehealth in the Philippines. *Acta Medica Philippina, 50*(4). https://doi.org/10.47895/amp.v50i4.763

Perrin, A., & Atske, S. (2021). Americans with disabilities less likely than those without to own some digital devices.

President's Advisory Commission on Consumer Protection and Quality in the Health Care Industry. (1998). *Quality first: Better health care for all Americans*. Advisory Commission on Consumer Protection and Quality in the Health Care Industry.

Rahimunnisa, K., Atchaiya, M., Arunachalam, B., & Divyaa, V. (2020). AI-based smart and intelligent wheelchair. *Journal of Applied Research and Technology, 18*(6), 362–367. https://doi.org/10.22201/icat.24486736e.2020.18.6.1351

Sahu, M., Grover, A., & Joshi, A. (2014). Role of mobile phone technology in health education in Asian and African countries: A systematic review. *International Journal of Electronic Healthcare, 7*(4), 269–286. https://doi.org/10.1504/IJEH.2014.064327

Scott, R. E., & Mars, M. (2015). Telehealth in the developing world: Current status and future prospects. *Smart Homecare Technology and TeleHealth, 25–37*,. https://doi.org/10.2147/SHTT.S75184

Senjam, S. S., & Manna, S. (2024). Assistive technology and disabilities in the context of sustainable developmental goals. In *The Palgrave encyclopedia of disability* (pp. 1–12). Springer Nature Switzerland. https://doi.org/10.1007/978-3-031-40858-8_67-1

Shanmugam, M., Shivakumar, V., Anitha, V., Meenapriya, B. P., Aishwarya, S., & Anitha, R. (2014). Behavioral pattern during dental pain in intellectually disabled children: A comparative study. *International Scholarly Research Notices, 2014*(1), Article 824125. https://doi.org/10.1155/2014/824125

Shin, P., Ku, L. C., Jones, E., & Rosenbaum, S. J. (2008). Analysis of the proposed rule on designation of medically underserved populations and health professional shortage areas.

Smith, C. A. (2019). Healthcare disparities in people with disabilities: Is there a cure? https://doi.org/10.14423/smj.0000000000000928

Sneha, M., Swetha, K., & Thilagavathy, A. (2022, December). AI-powered smart glasses for blind, deaf, and dumb. In *2022 5th International Conference on Advances in Science and Technology (ICAST)* (pp. 280–285). IEEE. https://doi.org/10.1109/ICAST55766.2022.10039557.

Stucki, G., Cieza, A., & Melvin, J. (2007). The international classification of functioning, disability and health: A unifying model for the conceptual description of the rehabilitation strategy. *Journal of Rehabilitation Medicine, 39*(4), 279–285. https://doi.org/10.2340/16501977-0041

Tang, L. Z. W., Ang, K. S., Amirul, M., Yusoff, M. B. M., Tng, C. K., Alyas, M. D. B. M., & Folianto, F. (2015, April). Augmented reality control home (ARCH) for disabled and elderlies. In *2015 IEEE Tenth international conference on intelligent sensors, sensor networks and information processing (ISSNIP)* (pp. 1–2). IEEE. https://doi.org/10.1109/ISSNIP.2015.7106975.

Umali, M. J. P. S., Evangelista-Sanchez, A. M. A., Lu, J. L., Ongkeko Jr, A. M., Sylim, P. G., Santos, A. D. F., & Pasco, P. M. D. (2016). Elaborating and discoursing the ethics in eHealth in the Philippines: Recommendations for health care practice and research. *Acta Medica Philippina, 50*(4). https://doi.org/10.47895/amp.v50i4.757

United States. Economics, Statistics Administration, United States. National Telecommunications, & Information Administration. (2000). *Falling through the net—Toward digital inclusion: A report on Americans' access to technology tools.* US Department of Commerce, Economic and Statistics Administration.

US Department of Health and Human Services. (2020). Office of disease prevention and health promotion. *Healthy People, 2010.*

Veerbeek, J. M., Langbroek-Amersfoort, A. C., Van Wegen, E. E., Meskers, C. G., & Kwakkel, G. (2017). Effects of robot-assisted therapy for the upper limb after stroke: A systematic review and meta-analysis. *Neurorehabilitation and Neural Repair, 31*(2), 107–121. https://doi.org/10.1177/1545968316666957

Villafania, J. (2018). Feasibility of telerehabilitation in the service delivery of speech-language pathology in the Philippines. In *Proceedings of the 11th Pan-Pacific Conference of Rehabilitation.*

Webster, P. (2020). Virtual health care in the era of COVID-19. *The Lancet, 395*(10231), 1180–1181. https://doi.org/10.1016/S0140-6736(20)30818-7

Wickramasinghe, N. (2008). An analysis of the healthcare informatics and systems in Southeast Asia: A current perspective from seven countries.

Wise, P. H. (2012). Emerging technologies and their impact on disability. *The Future of Children*, 169–191. http://www.jstor.org/stable/41475651

Chapter 5
Social Inclusion and Representation in Asian and African Continents

Abstract The focus on "inclusion" in the Sustainable Development Goals (SDGs) underscores the worldwide initiative to promote social, economic, and political integration among diverse groups of people. Despite progress in reducing extreme poverty, issues such as rising income inequality and the exclusion of vulnerable groups, including migrants, refugees, ethnic minorities, women, and people with disabilities, persist. In Africa, where approximately 15 percent of the population lives with disabilities, understanding the intersection of disability with factors such as gender, age, ethnicity, and socioeconomic status is critical for addressing the unique challenges faced by individuals with disabilities. The disability rights movement in Africa has grown significantly, advocating for greater inclusion and influencing policy decisions. Data collection on people with disabilities has provided valuable insights into the disparities they face, particularly in employment, education, and poverty. This chapter explores the concept of disability-inclusive development, which addresses the compounded discrimination that people with disabilities experience due to intersecting factors such as gender and ethnicity. Focusing on key areas like inclusive education, employment, healthcare, and accessibility, the twin-track approach to disability-inclusive development ensures that people with disabilities are active participants and beneficiaries in the development process. This approach is essential to ending extreme poverty and promoting social inclusion while also highlighting the need for context-specific strategies to address the diverse needs of individuals with disabilities across regions. Through a multifaceted approach that combines global commitments with local solutions, the chapter underscores the importance of disability-inclusive development in creating equitable opportunities for all.

Keywords Inclusion · Sustainable Development Goals · Disabilities · Poverty · Advocacy

5.1 Introduction

The emphasis on inclusion in the Sustainable Development Goals (SDGs) reflects the global push for social, economic, and political integration across diverse populations. While significant progress has been made in reducing extreme poverty, other challenges persist, including rising income inequality, the impacts of the Great Recession, and the exclusion of vulnerable groups such as migrants, refugees, ethnic minorities, women, and people with disabilities. These issues are compounded by spatial and social disparities, where the benefits and costs of globalization are unevenly distributed across regions and communities. The demand for equal rights, political inclusion, and access to essential services has intensified as democratization and liberalization have exposed persistent inequities. The exclusionary effects of economic and political pressures, including discrimination in hiring, housing, and social services, have led to widespread social movements advocating for equal treatment and recognition. Addressing social inclusion, therefore, requires global commitments and context-specific solutions. Local place and institutional configurations significantly shape opportunities, identity, and access to resources, meaning that these factors must be considered when crafting inclusive strategies (Silver, 2015). Fig 5.1 represents the concept of Social Inclusion for individuals with disabilities through a circular flow of key elements.

In Africa, around 15 percent of the population lives with disabilities, a statistic that mirrors global trends. Addressing the needs of individuals with disabilities in the region requires a nuanced understanding of how factors such as the type and severity of disability, gender, age, location, ethnicity, sexual orientation, gender identity, marital status, and socioeconomic status intersect. These intersecting factors can create advantages or amplify disadvantages more often. The disability rights movement in Africa has emerged as one of the most dynamic social movements on the continent today. With the guiding principle of "nothing for us without us," the movement has influenced government budget decisions and research priorities, raised awareness, and helped reduce the stigma surrounding people with disabilities. Additionally, the advocacy for albinism is growing, further adding to the importance of disability rights in the African context. Advocacy has significantly contributed to the availability of data and analysis, which, in turn, strengthens the efforts of these movements (Das & Espinoza, 2019; United Nations, 2006).

In several African countries, the collection of data on people with disabilities has enabled a more empirical focus on the adverse outcomes faced by this group. Studies have shown that people with disabilities are more likely to work in self-employment within agriculture and are less likely to be formally employed in the traditional job market. Employment outcomes vary significantly depending on the type and intensity of the disability. For instance, a study using data from Ethiopia, Malawi, Tanzania, and Uganda found the most significant disparities in Tanzania, where only 53 percent of individuals with severe functional difficulties were employed, compared to 85 percent of individuals without such challenges. The complex relationship between disability

5.1 Introduction

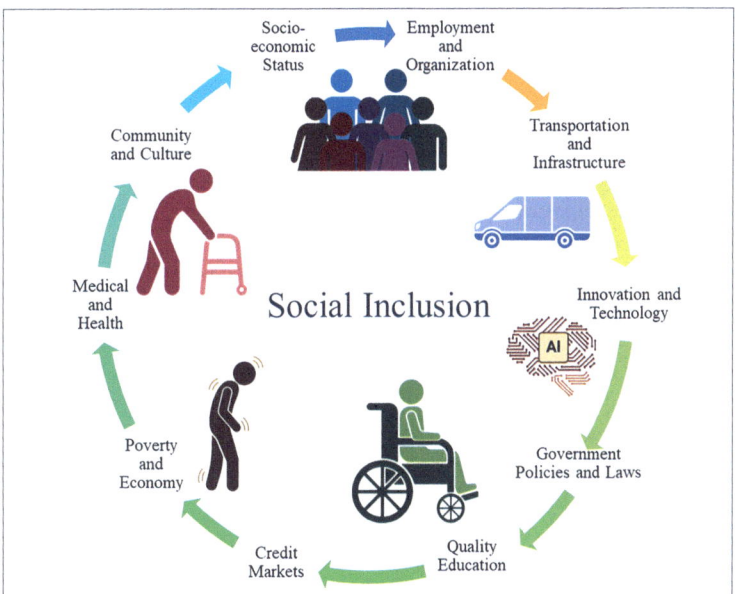

Fig. 5.1 Concept of social inclusion for individuals with disabilities (It highlights community participation, emphasizing integrating people with disabilities into society. Accessible transportation is depicted as a crucial factor in ensuring mobility through adapted vehicles. The role of AI in assistive technology is also showcased, demonstrating how AI-powered innovations enhance accessibility and independence. Additionally, the image includes wheelchair accessibility, underscoring the importance of inclusive infrastructure. It also acknowledges neurological and motor disabilities, representing the challenges faced by individuals with movement disorders. Furthermore, elderly and mobility support are depicted through assistive devices like walkers, catering to seniors and individuals with limited mobility)

and poverty is also notable: while persons with disabilities make up a disproportionately large share of people experiencing poverty, not all individuals with disabilities are impoverished. Moreover, there is significant evidence showing lower levels of educational attainment among people with disabilities in Africa. When disability status intersects with gender, the disadvantages become even more pronounced, as women with disabilities face additional barriers to education, employment, and social participation. Moreover, outcomes vary depending on the type of disability, yet the lack of reliable data remains a significant obstacle to further analysis and intervention. For example, data on individuals with intellectual disabilities is particularly scarce, as are services available to support this group of individuals (Rehman et al., 2022).

In Asia, ending extreme poverty requires incorporating disability-inclusive development, much like in other regions. Disability-inclusive development recognizes and addresses the intersection of disability with different forms of discrimination, such as gender, ethnicity, religion, age, and national or social origin, which can compound exclusion and disadvantage. Disability-inclusive development ensures that people with disabilities are considered beneficiaries and actively included in development processes as participants. This approach is carried out through multilateral and multi-sectoral partnerships involving governments, development banks, the private sector, and civil society. These partnerships raise awareness and maximize impact by aligning efforts across industries. Disability inclusion can be mainstreamed across institutions or implemented in targeted programs and projects. The latter is part of what is known as the twin-track approach, which combines these two strategies to create inclusive and effective development. This twin-track approach follows a multi-sectoral and life-cycle framework, with a focus on key areas such as early childhood development, inclusive education, community-based development, supported independent living, employment, economic empowerment, active aging, inclusive social protection, and the availability of affordable healthcare and assistive technologies (Kidd, 2013). Children with cognitive impairments often depend on their caregivers to understand and interpret their signs of distress (Shanmugam et al., 2014). Improving accessibility is also a central focus, including access to transport, urban environments, information and communication technologies, water, and social services.

Additionally, the approach emphasizes the importance of inclusive emergency preparedness and response to ensure that people with disabilities are considered in crises. Furthermore, there is a strong emphasis on improving data and information regarding individuals with disabilities, which is crucial for making informed policy decisions and implementing targeted interventions (Kidd, 2013). Achieving inclusive development that addresses the needs of people with disabilities is essential to ending extreme poverty and ensuring equitable opportunities for all. The intersectionality of disability with other forms of discrimination highlights the complexity of exclusion, necessitating a multifaceted approach that combines global commitments with context-specific solutions. This chapter explores the critical role of disability-inclusive development in addressing the global challenge of extreme poverty and fostering social, economic, and political integration for all populations. It examines how the intersection of disability with factors such as gender, ethnicity, age, and socioeconomic status can amplify exclusion and disadvantage, particularly for vulnerable groups like women, ethnic minorities, refugees, and people with disabilities.

5.2 Disability in Media, Arts, and Sports

There are currently 650 million people with disabilities worldwide, with 450 million living in the global south. As the largest and most marginalized minority group, people with disabilities face pervasive prejudice, discrimination, and poverty. Despite the progress made in disability rights, they continue to experience exclusion, stigma, and underemployment. Sport, however, has become a powerful tool in challenging societal stereotypes and highlighting the abilities of people with disabilities. In 2006, the UN Convention on the Rights of Persons with Disabilities marked a pivotal moment in this struggle by recognizing the right of people with disabilities to engage in sport, physical activity, and recreation, mainly through Article 30. This shift moved away from a medical, charity-based view of disability and embraced a rights-based approach, emphasizing inclusion and equal access (Gerbrandt, 2009).

However, despite these advancements in disability rights, the literature on disability sports remains disproportionately focused on experiences from the global north, often overlooking the realities faced by the majority of people with disabilities in the global south. Disability impacts nearly 10% of the global working-age population, and 40% of people over 65 experience some form of disability (Braithwaite & Mont, 2009). Yet, many countries, especially in the global south, lack accurate national disability data, and disability is frequently overlooked in global poverty assessments (Babalola & Daniel Olatunde, 2012). Consequently, people with disabilities often find themselves subjected to stigma, exclusion, and underemployment. The United Nations' Millennium Development Goals (MDGs), which focused on eradicating extreme poverty, did not explicitly address disability, but their focus on poverty disproportionately affected disabled individuals (Le Clair, 2011). These individuals face systemic discrimination, with many subjected to abuse and social ostracism (Marucha & Ngigi, 2018). For example, a Kenyan student reported being physically punished by teachers for being late due to his wheelchair (Le Clair, 2009), while a Canadian Paralympian was ostracized by children who were unfamiliar with his disability. Such experiences highlight the deeply ingrained discriminatory attitudes that continue to prevail. While efforts to challenge these attitudes have had some success (Le Clair, 2012), complete societal change is still a long way off. Global initiatives like Terry Fox's Marathon of Hope and Rick Hansen's Man in Motion World Tour have utilized physical activity to raise awareness, challenge stereotypes, and support the inclusion of disabled individuals. These efforts, along with the work of many disability sports advocates, challenge the assumptions about disability and limitations. The demand for representation and inclusion is central to these initiatives, a struggle that James Charlton articulates in *Nothing About Us Without Us*, highlighting the ongoing battle against paternalism and exclusion. Despite some progress, disabled individuals remain significantly underrepresented, particularly in academic discourse, underscoring the need for continued advocacy and systemic change (Kasum et al., 2011).

Combat sports, in particular, have the potential to offer profound benefits to individuals with disabilities. These sports can help improve physical health, mental focus, emotional well-being, and overall resilience. By making minimal adjustments to rules and equipment, many combat sports are becoming increasingly accessible to people with disabilities. These activities help develop motor skills, reduce stress and depression, and promote essential life skills such as responsibility, discipline, respect, aggression management, and cooperation. While the benefits of combat sports may take longer to manifest compared to activities like walking or swimming, they offer a unique and powerful way to foster resilience and coping skills that help individuals with disabilities navigate daily life challenges. Furthermore, including combat sports in broader fitness programs has enhanced their appeal and effectiveness for the general population and people with disabilities (Dragojlović et al., 2009).

In Serbia, where combat sports are currently underrepresented among individuals with disabilities, integrating these sports into existing national federations and combat clubs for non-disabled athletes represents a practical solution. These clubs already have the infrastructure and resources necessary for training, and national federations handle legal and organizational aspects. Educating coaches and athletes on how to train people with disabilities, sports clubs, and federations can rapidly expand access to combat sports for this underserved group. This shift will likely result in significant growth in the quantity and quality of participation in combat sports for people with disabilities. As participation grows, the visibility and popularity of disability-inclusive sports clubs and federations will increase, raising their profile and providing potential financial benefits through enhanced media coverage and broader representation. In turn, this could improve the overall quality of life for individuals with disabilities, making combat sports a valuable and accessible option for individuals and national sports organizations (Guan & Hong, 2016).

The development of disability sports in China offers a compelling example of how systematic and structured approaches can foster talent and improve participation. In the 1980s, disability sports in China lacked a formal training system, making athlete selection challenging. However, by 1992, the China Disabled Persons Federation (CDPF) had developed disability sports, established specialized organizations, and employed full-time staff. The CDPF implemented a pyramid training and selection system similar to that used for non-disabled athletes, identifying young talent through provincial games and training camps focused on basic skills. Athletes selected for provincial teams undergo semi-professional training, and the most promising athletes are chosen for national teams, where they receive intensive training for the Paralympic Games. This multi-level system supports athletes' progression from local to national teams and is part of China's "whole country support for elite sport" approach, which has significantly improved Chinese athletes' success at the Paralympics (Le Roux, 2018).

Disability arts, as a dynamic form of community expression, intersect with disability sports in ways that reflect broader social movements for equality and inclusion. Disability arts, often seen as a form of protest against oppressive social models, also highlight the personal and experiential aspects of disability. According to Cameron (2016), disability arts should be understood within the context of the disabled people's movement, which continues to push for equality and recognition. In the UK, the disability arts movement has been diverse and inclusive, with artists such as Mat Fraser and the Candoco Dance Company showcasing innovative performances. Similarly, the Die Schlumper collective has been active in Germany since 1985, benefiting from sponsorships that enable full-time professional participation. Stöckl, 2015 emphasizes that all art forms reflect a complex social world and that art transcends the artist's intent to evoke deep emotional and cognitive responses in the viewer. Drawing on Gell's (1998) anthropology of art, Stöckl highlights that art objects possess agency, influencing both the artist and the viewer by creating powerful atmospheres that generate emotional reactions (Gell, 1998; Le Roux, 2018; Stöckl, 2015).

Therefore, combat sports, disability sports, and disability arts all play crucial roles in challenging the societal stigma and discrimination that people with disabilities face. These movements, whether through physical activity or artistic expression, help foster inclusion, promote equal rights, and advocate for representation. As these fields grow, they offer powerful tools to combat exclusion and advance the cause of disability rights globally.

While the global movement for disability rights, inclusive sports, and disability arts continues progressing, significant regional differences remain, particularly between Asia and Africa. In Asia, countries like China have developed well-organized systems for disability sports, with government-led initiatives such as the China Disabled Persons Federation (CDPF) creating robust pathways for athletes with disabilities to progress from local to national teams. This structured approach has contributed to China's success in the Paralympics and has fostered a more comprehensive recognition of disability sports. Additionally, disability arts in Asia, particularly in countries like Japan and South Korea, are increasingly being integrated into mainstream cultural movements, benefiting from state support and institutionalized frameworks for artistic expression.

In contrast, Africa faces more pronounced challenges in terms of infrastructure, data collection, and funding. While there are notable examples of disability sports and arts in some African nations, such as establishing national Paralympic committees and growing grassroots movements, the continent still lacks the comprehensive national systems and institutional frameworks seen in parts of Asia. Access to disability-inclusive sports is often limited due to financial constraints, lack of awareness, and the absence of trained personnel. Similarly, the disability arts movement in Africa is still in its nascent stages, with many artists facing difficulties gaining recognition and support for their work.

Moreover, in both regions, stigma and discrimination against people with disabilities remain pervasive, but the social and cultural context varies. In Asia, particularly in rural areas, traditional attitudes toward disability can be deeply ingrained, though there is a growing push for inclusion through public awareness campaigns and media representation. In Africa, the social model of disability, which emphasizes inclusion and rights, is still gaining traction in many regions, with disability often being seen through a medical or charity lens.

Ultimately, while both Asia and Africa have made significant strides in promoting the rights and inclusion of people with disabilities, the level of progress and institutional support varies significantly. Asia, particularly countries like China, have more established systems in place for both disability sports and arts, while Africa faces more systemic challenges but has a growing movement driven by grassroots efforts. Continued advocacy, improved infrastructure, and international collaboration will be key to bridging these gaps and ensuring that people with disabilities, regardless of region, can fully participate in sports, arts, and society (Jodell & Bian, 2023).

5.3 Advocacy Movements and Leadership by Young Activists

Civic engagement is fundamental to a democracy, ensuring that it truly reflects "the people." However, people with disabilities face significant systemic challenges that hinder their full participation in democratic life. People with disabilities who are also people of color face further obstacles, as research consistently indicates that people of color often have limited access to education, health, and employment opportunities. This exclusion leads to their underrepresentation in civic life, where discussions and efforts that impact disabled people are often dominated by the voices of white, non-disabled individuals, reinforcing a systemic imbalance of power (Ho et al., 2020).

The exclusion of disabled individuals from meaningful civic engagement has created an environment where their participation remains fragmented and ableist. As a result, disabled people experience marginalization that limits their ability to influence social, economic, and political progress. Despite ongoing efforts to engage people with disabilities in civic participation and leadership, these initiatives often fail to reflect the lived experiences of disabled individuals, leaving their voices unheard. To address these disparities, sustained representation and leadership from disabled people are crucial within and outside traditional democratic processes. A genuinely democratic system requires allyship and relationship-building across movements and sectors. Philanthropy is key in supporting disability-led efforts to challenge ableism and increase disabled people's influence over policies, systems, and structures that directly affect them (Berghs et al., 2020).

Neoliberalism, austerity measures, climate change, and the rise of far-right movements have intensified the challenges facing disabled people globally, leading to an increase in impairments and deaths, as well as the erosion of disability rights. These external challenges have left institutions and organizations struggling to respond effectively. However, disabled people and their allies continue to resist through various forms of activism, including mass protests, artistic movements, and digital activism like Black Lives Matter and MeToo. Social media has democratized activism, providing a global platform for engagement. Yet, criticisms of "clicktivism" and the commercialization of activism have emerged, highlighting the limitations of digital movements. Despite these concerns, disability activism remains underrepresented and often framed narrowly around rights and individual identities, overlooking the broader social and political implications of disability. In response, urgent calls for disability justice are emerging, calling for a more inclusive and intersectional approach to activism that considers the varied and complex challenges disabled people face (Watermeyer, 2006).

In particular, young activists in Asia and Africa have become powerful voices in disability rights advocacy. These youth leaders challenge societal norms and fight for greater inclusion and policy changes to ensure better access to education, healthcare, employment, and social participation for people with disabilities. In Asia, countries such as India, Pakistan, and the Philippines have seen a surge of young activists

5.3 Advocacy Movements and Leadership by Young Activists

leveraging digital platforms to raise awareness on accessibility, discrimination, and the right to a dignified life. Similarly, in Africa, youth-led movements in nations like Kenya, Nigeria, and South Africa are essential in promoting disability rights, focusing on improving infrastructure, legal protections, and social integration for disabled individuals. These young leaders, many of whom have disabilities themselves, are reshaping the global conversation about disability, not just advocating for policy change but also challenging societal stigma. Their activism is pivotal in building more inclusive and equitable societies for people with disabilities across these regions (Katsui, 2005).

In South Africa, the history of the disability rights movement is closely tied to the experiences of disabled people under apartheid, shaped by multiple forces and organizations. Under apartheid, disabled people's lives were marked by the broader inequalities of South African society, with black disabled individuals facing additional hardships due to poverty, violence, and deprivation. However, all disabled people, regardless of race, suffered from discrimination and marginalization, with limited access to fundamental rights such as education, employment, and health services. These struggles laid the foundation for creating Disabled People's South Africa (DPSA) in 1984. As the largest cross-disability organization in the country, DPSA has played a crucial role in advocating for the rights of disabled individuals. The founders of DPSA believed that disabled people's liberation required not only the end of apartheid but also a shift in how disability was understood. This meant moving away from the view that disabled people were dependent and powerless, a shift that shaped the disability rights movement into a struggle against both apartheid and societal attitudes toward disability (Finkelstein, 1980).

In Central Asia, the disability rights movement is heavily influenced by the region's legacy as part of the Soviet Union. Under the Soviet regime, disabled people were labeled as "invalids" and excluded from the workforce, as workability was central to the regime's ideology. This medicalized view of disability led to a system that isolated disabled people from society, making them essentially invisible. Even after gaining independence, many Central Asian governments continued to perpetuate these practices, treating disability as an individual issue rather than a societal one shaped by discrimination and inaccessibility. These attitudes persist in current government policies, leaving disabled people without access to essential services such as education, employment, and social rights. The introduction of market economies further marginalized disabled individuals, as the competition in these new economies was often beyond their reach. As a result, disabled people in Central Asia remain excluded from many aspects of society, with few opportunities to challenge their status (Lawson & Beckett, 2021).

The marginalization of disabled people in Central Asia is not only institutional but also psychological. Prevailing governmental attitudes have fostered a sense of inferiority and passivity among disabled individuals. Prejudices are widespread, impacting their daily interactions and relationships. This social isolation leads to dependency, as many disabled people internalize the view that they are abnormal and deviant. The physical and psychological barriers created by government policies make it difficult for disabled individuals to challenge their marginalization, further limiting their integration into society. A lack of infrastructure, education, employment opportunities, and essential equipment compounds these challenges. Disabled people's organizations (DPOs) in the region are few and often poorly equipped, relying on international funding and adopting a charity-based model rather than a rights-based advocacy approach (UNICEF, 2018).

While the social model of disability provides valuable insights into the challenges faced by disabled people in Central Asia, it needs to be adapted to reflect regional differences. The experience of disability in the region is shaped by collective societal factors as well as the unique personal experiences of disabled individuals. A one-size-fits-all approach is inadequate for addressing these challenges. The rise of NGOs in the disability sector, including government-supported (GONGOs) and international organizations, has not led to meaningful change for disabled people in the region. Despite the growing number of NGOs, many of these organizations fail to meet the actual needs of disabled individuals, with their activities remaining inaccessible or irrelevant. These systemic issues highlight the need for a comprehensive, rights-based approach to disability advocacy and activism that is locally informed and better supports the needs of disabled people in Central Asia (Durham et al., 2013).

The urgent need marks the global disability rights movement for inclusive, intersectional activism that centers on the lived experiences of disabled people across all regions. Whether in the context of South Africa's apartheid history, Central Asia's Soviet legacy, or the rising youth-led movements in Asia and Africa, the struggle for disability rights continues to evolve. Overcoming systemic barriers, challenging societal stigma, and ensuring sustained representation are key to achieving meaningful change and creating more inclusive societies for people with disabilities.

5.4 Disability in Conflict Zones and Humanitarian Crises

Disability in conflict zones and humanitarian crises remains among the most under-researched and overlooked issues in global development and human rights advocacy. The effects of war, natural disasters, and humanitarian emergencies on persons with disabilities are multifaceted and devastating, exacerbating existing inequalities and leaving individuals and communities vulnerable to further harm. In regions such as Asia and Africa, where political instability, armed conflict, and environmental disasters frequently occur, the disabled population often faces disproportionate challenges in terms of physical, social, and economic security.

The intersection of disability and conflict is a hidden crisis that significantly worsens the vulnerability of disabled individuals, particularly in Asia and Africa. Armed conflict, often characterized by violent acts such as bombings, landmines, and armed violence directly leads to new impairments, including amputations, spinal cord injuries, and traumatic brain injuries. The long-term effects of these injuries create a new class of disabled individuals who would not have been disabled under normal circumstances. Additionally, those who already live with disabilities are subjected to even more violence, deprivation, and displacement than their non-disabled counterparts. Countries such as Afghanistan, Syria, Sudan, and Somalia have seen staggering numbers of new disabilities as a result of armed conflict, with a significant proportion of the disabled population comprising individuals who sustained life-altering injuries during the conflict (Tyler, 2021).

In war-torn regions like Myanmar and Afghanistan, disability rates are notably higher due to the widespread presence of landmines and explosive remnants of war (ERWs). These devices cause severe injuries, particularly to civilians, who are often left without adequate medical treatment in remote or underdeveloped areas. According to the Landmine and Cluster Munition Monitor, over 1,500 people in Afghanistan alone have been killed or maimed by landmines since 2018, with many of these victims suffering long-term disabilities (Cathcart, 2016; Dukhan, 2016; Tyler, 2021). Similarly, in conflict zones like South Sudan and the Central African Republic (CAR), access to healthcare is minimal, meaning that many disabled people are denied the rehabilitation and medical support they desperately need to regain mobility or improve their quality of life (Reilly, 2010).

Displacement is another devastating consequence of conflict for disabled individuals. Forced migration amplifies their difficulties, whether within a country or across borders. Refugees and internally displaced persons (IDPs) often end up in overcrowded camps or informal settlements, where the infrastructure is woefully inadequate and essential services are limited. These areas typically lack the physical accessibility necessary for people with disabilities, such as ramps, accessible toilets, and safe spaces. As a result, disabled individuals are often confined to tents, unable to access food, healthcare, or other essential services (Cook & Ne, 2018). For instance, in the camps in Bangladesh housing Rohingya refugees fleeing persecution in Myanmar, disabled persons face severe challenges in accessing healthcare, education, and livelihood opportunities. At the same time, many are at an increased risk of violence and abuse, as reported by the United Nations High Commissioner for Refugees (UNHCR) (Barbareschi et al., 2021).

In conflict zones, social stigma, discrimination, and exclusion are all too common for disabled individuals. Disabilities are often associated with shame, leading to the marginalization of people with impairments in the broader social fabric. This social stigma makes it even harder for disabled individuals to participate in humanitarian relief efforts, rendering them invisible in recovery processes. They are often viewed as "burdens," incapable of contributing to rebuilding their communities, which further limits their access to resources and opportunities in these fragile environments (Rohwerder, 2013). This exclusion from society and decision-making processes worsens their isolation and deepens the inequalities they face.

The humanitarian response to disability in crisis zones is often inadequate and insufficient. While international humanitarian organizations, governments, and NGOs have made strides toward recognizing the need for disability inclusion, it remains a low priority in many crisis settings. Humanitarian aid is typically designed with the assumption that all individuals can equally access and benefit from it, which is rarely the case when considering the specific needs of disabled persons (Mirza, 2011). Accessibility remains a significant barrier in many humanitarian settings. For example, infrastructure in refugee camps and informal settlements is almost always designed for able-bodied individuals, leaving those with disabilities at a disadvantage when trying to access even essential services such as food distribution, healthcare, and sanitation. Distribution points for food, water, and medical aid are often inaccessible for people who rely on mobility aids like wheelchairs, crutches, or prosthetic limbs (McBride-Henry et al., 2023).

Furthermore, persons with disabilities have specific health needs that are often overlooked in emergency health interventions. These needs include specialized rehabilitation services, mobility aids, mental health support, and other medical treatments. In many crises, health systems are overwhelmed and under-resourced, making it challenging to address these unique requirements (Harris & Enfield, 2003). The lack of adequate services for disabled individuals not only exacerbates their physical and mental health problems but also leads to long-term disadvantages in post-crisis recovery.

One of the key factors for improving the humanitarian response to disability in conflict zones is the active involvement of disabled individuals in the design and implementation of aid interventions. Historically, disabled people have been treated as passive recipients of aid rather than active participants in decision-making processes. The "Nothing About Us Without Us" principle, which advocates for the inclusion of disabled people at all levels of decision-making, has gained traction in humanitarian circles, yet its implementation remains inconsistent. In practice, this means ensuring that disability is considered in planning refugee camps, food distribution, and developing education and healthcare services. Disabled individuals must be involved in shaping policies and programs to ensure their needs are met effectively (Martínez-Medina et al., 2022).

International frameworks, such as the CRPD and the Sendai Framework for Disaster Risk Reduction, have underscored the importance of ensuring that disabled people have access to humanitarian aid and are included in disaster preparedness and recovery efforts. However, implementing these frameworks remains challenging due to a lack of data on disability, insufficient training for humanitarian workers, and limited resources for inclusive programming (Bou-Karroum et al., 2020). Despite these challenges, these frameworks provide a foundation for improving the inclusion of disabled people in humanitarian responses.

The impact of conflict and humanitarian crises on disabled individuals extends well beyond the immediate harm caused. In post-crisis settings, disabled individuals often face ongoing difficulties in rebuilding their lives and reintegrating into society. Post-crisis recovery requires a shift from emergency relief to long-term rehabilitation and recovery, which includes addressing issues such as economic empowerment, healthcare, education, and social inclusion (Louw et al., 2021). Rehabilitation services, including access to prosthetics, physical therapy, and psychological support, are critical for disabled people to regain their independence and quality of life. Unfortunately, in many conflict zones, these services are either unavailable or inadequate, leaving many disabled individuals without the support they need (Valenti, 2022).

Economic empowerment programs for disabled individuals are also rare, and many disabled people find themselves excluded from livelihood programs. This exclusion further exacerbates their vulnerability and dependence on external aid. Moreover, displaced children with disabilities often face barriers to education, including physical inaccessibility, lack of specialized support, and social stigma. Even as educational infrastructure is rebuilt in post-crisis settings, disabled children remain at risk of being excluded from schooling, which undermines their potential for future success (Disability U. N., 2018).

Social inclusion remains a significant challenge in post-conflict societies. Disabled individuals often struggle to reintegrate into their communities, facing both physical and social barriers that prevent them from participating fully in social and economic life. Rebuilding inclusive communities requires addressing the infrastructure barriers and the social stigmas perpetuating discrimination. A more inclusive approach to community rebuilding would ensure that disabled people can lead independent lives and contribute meaningfully to reconstructing their societies.

Disability in conflict zones and humanitarian crises across Asia and Africa is an urgent issue that requires more attention and action from the international community. Disabled individuals face a myriad of challenges, including physical barriers, social stigma, limited access to healthcare, and exclusion from humanitarian aid and recovery efforts. To improve the situation, it is essential to prioritize disability-inclusive humanitarian assistance by ensuring that interventions are accessible and responsive to the needs of disabled people. Active participation of disabled individuals in decision-making processes, reliable data collection, and long-term recovery programs that include rehabilitation and economic empowerment are all critical for ensuring that disabled individuals are not left behind as communities rebuild after crises and conflicts. Table 5.1 highlights key global disability rights issues, focusing on civic engagement, intersectionality, and policy advocacy.

5.5 Building an Inclusive Society: Pathways Forward

Disability inclusion remains one of the most pressing challenges globally, with significant implications for nations in Asia and Africa. Over 1 billion people worldwide live with some form of disability, the majority of whom reside in low- and middle-income countries, especially in the Global South. In regions such as Asia and Africa, individuals with disabilities often face systemic marginalization due to a complex combination of stigmatization, inadequate infrastructure, limited healthcare access, and barriers to education and employment. Achieving an inclusive society entails ensuring that individuals with disabilities are integrated and actively participate in the societal, cultural, economic, and political spheres. This requires dismantling physical, social, and cultural barriers and ensuring equitable access to education, healthcare, employment, and civic life. Moreover, fostering a shift in societal attitudes toward disability is essential for creating a genuinely inclusive environment (Sen, 2000).

In Asia and Africa, social exclusion and marginalization are deeply entrenched issues that undermine social cohesion and economic development. While particular

Table 5.1 Global disability rights issues, focusing on civic engagement, intersectionality, and policy advocacy

Key Issues	Specific Areas	Action to be taken
Barriers to Civic Engagement	Global	Ensure better accessibility for disabled individuals in democratic processes Advocate for systemic changes that remove education, health, and employment barriers
Exclusion of Disabled People of Color	Global	Address racial and disability exclusion through targeted policies Promote racial and disability intersectionality in civic life and leadership
Fragmented Civic Participation	Global	Establish inclusive platforms that amplify disabled voices Foster leadership opportunities for disabled people within civic institutions
Global Challenges (Neoliberalism, Austerity)	Global	Push for policies that protect disability rights in the face of economic austerity Strengthen protections against the erosion of disability rights due to global political movements (e.g., far-right, climate change)
Digital Activism and Its Limitations	Global	Improve the accessibility and inclusivity of digital activism platforms for disabled people Ensure that digital movements are backed by real-world actions that drive substantial change
Disability Justice and Intersectionality	Global	Build coalitions across movements to address both disability and other social justice issues Focus on both individual and collective disability rights, emphasizing the interconnectedness of issues like poverty, race, and gender
Youth-Led Disability Movements	Asia, Africa	Support youth-led movements by providing platforms and resources for advocacy Ensure that youth activists are involved in policy development and decision-making processes
South Africa's Disability Movement	South Africa	Promote policies that address both apartheid's legacy and the ongoing marginalization of disabled people Strengthen the leadership of organizations like DPSA and other local DPOs in advocating for disability rights
Central Asia's Disability Challenges	Central Asia	Advocate for a shift from medicalized views of disability to a rights-based approach Push for comprehensive disability-inclusive legislation and infrastructure development Promote local advocacy organizations (DPOs) to adopt a rights-based model rather than charity-based approaches
Global Disability Rights Movement	Global	Ensure that disability rights activism is intersectional, including voices from all regions, backgrounds, and disabilities Build long-term cross-sector alliances to address systemic barriers and ensure sustainable change for disabled people worldwide

5.5 Building an Inclusive Society: Pathways Forward

strides have been made in these regions, the path to building truly inclusive societies is complex and multifaceted. A genuinely inclusive society involves integrating marginalized groups and providing equitable opportunities for all citizens regardless of race, ethnicity, gender, religion, disability, or socioeconomic status. This is crucial for reducing inequality, fostering social stability, and promoting collective prosperity. The challenge, however, lies in addressing historical, cultural, and systemic barriers that have long perpetuated exclusion. In these regions, factors such as the legacies of colonialism, ethnic divisions, political marginalization, gender inequality, and economic disparities present significant obstacles to achieving social inclusion. Hence, building an inclusive society requires transformative strategies across various levels, including legal, political, financial, and cultural (Kabeer, 2005).

Social exclusion in both Asia and Africa arises from a complex web of historical, political, and socioeconomic factors. Ethnic, religious, and regional inequalities are particularly stark in these regions, making it difficult for minority groups to access essential services such as education, healthcare, and economic opportunities. Entrenched stereotypes and cultural biases often compound these disparities, further marginalizing already disadvantaged communities (Bhattacharjee, 2024). Ethnic and religious tensions are significant drivers of exclusion in both Asia and Africa. In Southeast Asia, for example, the Rohingya crisis in Myanmar demonstrates how ethnic minorities can be systematically deprived of citizenship and fundamental rights, leaving them vulnerable to violence and displacement (Irobi, 2005). Similarly, ethnic divisions in Sub-Saharan Africa often lead to violent conflicts, marginalizing certain groups politically and economically and deepening social and economic inequalities (Dahal et al., 2022). These historical and political factors create barriers to access, perpetuating cycles of poverty and marginalization.

Gender inequality plays a central role in social exclusion across both continents. In many African and Asian countries, women, especially those in rural areas, face significant challenges in accessing education, healthcare, and economic opportunities. Cultural and traditional practices often restrict their participation in decision-making processes and limit their rights to property and inheritance, further entrenching their disenfranchisement. This affects their social mobility and inhibits broader societal progress, as women's exclusion from contributing fully to the economy and governance diminishes overall societal development (Dahal et al., 2022; Nasrabadi et al., 2024).

Economic inequality is another fundamental driver of exclusion. Widespread income inequality, unequal access to quality jobs, and the unequal distribution of resources such as land and housing have created a significant divide between the rich and the poor. Marginalized communities are often relegated to impoverished living conditions with limited access to essential services like healthcare, education, and financial resources. This lack of opportunity perpetuates cycles of poverty, leaving these communities with few prospects for advancement. The absence of social safety nets and economic empowerment mechanisms further exacerbates these challenges, trapping marginalized groups in a state of persistent exclusion. Political exclusion remains a significant issue, where marginalized groups are often underrepresented in political processes. In many countries, weak governance, corruption, and a lack of political will hinder the effective implementation of inclusive policies. Rural and urban marginalized communities often lack a voice in legislative and governance processes, further entrenching their exclusion. Political underrepresentation also weakens democratic institutions and hinders the development of inclusive laws and policies (DESA, 2009).

Addressing the structural barriers perpetuating exclusion, discrimination, and inequality in Asia and Africa requires comprehensive strategies involving legal reforms, political representation, economic empowerment, and equitable access to education. Overcoming these barriers will contribute to social cohesion and bolster national development. Effective legislation is foundational in creating inclusive societies. Legal frameworks that protect marginalized groups, including ethnic minorities, women, people with disabilities, and economically disadvantaged populations, are essential to guarantee equal opportunities and safeguard against discrimination. In countries like India, affirmative action policies, including reservations for marginalized communities in education and employment, have been introduced to address historical inequalities. Such measures aim to give these groups the necessary opportunities to uplift themselves socially and economically. However, the success of such reforms depends on the effective enforcement and implementation of these laws (Cordenillo & Gardes, 2013).

Political inclusion is another key pillar in building inclusive societies. Ensuring that political decision-making processes reflect the diversity of the population is crucial for fostering inclusion. This requires increasing the political participation of underrepresented groups through electoral reforms, quotas, and capacity-building initiatives. A notable example is Rwanda, where gender equality in politics has been a significant success. Women hold more than 60% of parliamentary seats, making Rwanda a global leader in gender inclusivity in governance. This high level of female representation has led to the creation of policies addressing women's issues, such as maternal healthcare and gender-based violence (Chu & Gupta, 1998).

Economic empowerment is essential to break the cycles of poverty and exclusion. Marginalized communities often lack access to financial resources, employment opportunities, and economic support systems. Thus, creating avenues for economic inclusion is crucial for social cohesion and long-term stability. Microfinance initiatives in countries like Bangladesh have effectively enabled women and low-income populations to start small businesses and achieve financial independence. Furthermore, governments must establish social safety nets, such as cash transfers, subsidized healthcare, and unemployment benefits, to protect vulnerable populations from economic shocks (Spatafora, 2021).

Education remains one of the most powerful tools for fostering social mobility and creating long-term equity. Quality education empowers individuals to actively participate in life's economic, political, and social spheres. Despite progress in increasing enrollment rates in primary and secondary schools, marginalized groups, especially those from rural areas, ethnic minorities, and girls, still face significant barriers to education. Cultural norms, poverty, and inadequate infrastructure prevent these groups from accessing quality education. Governments and NGOs must invest in inclusive education programs, build infrastructure, and eliminate gender-specific educational barriers. Initiatives to change social attitudes about the value of education for girls can also effectively overcome cultural resistance (Spiel et al., 2018).

Building inclusive societies in Asia and Africa requires a multifaceted and transformative approach. Legislative reforms, political representation, economic empowerment, and education must address the historical, social, and cultural factors contributing to exclusion. Governments, civil society, international organizations, and local communities must collaborate to create inclusive environments that provide equal opportunities for all citizens. Achieving inclusivity is about creating opportunities for marginalized groups and recognizing that their full participation in society contributes to national development, stability, and prosperity. Through collective action and commitment to social justice, Asia and Africa can create societies where all individuals, regardless of their background, have the opportunity to thrive and contribute to the collective well-being of their nations.

5.6 Conclusion

Building inclusive societies for people with disabilities in Asia and Africa requires a transformative approach addressing systemic barriers, societal stigma, and historical injustices. While progress has been made in some areas, particularly in disability sports in Asia and grassroots movements in Africa, significant regional disparities persist. The chapter highlights the urgent need for a multi-pronged strategy encompassing (1) Strengthening disability-inclusive development frameworks, focusing on access to education, healthcare, and employment; (2) Investing in infrastructure and data collection to inform effective interventions; (3) Promoting inclusive, intersectional activism led by disabled individuals themselves, particularly in addressing the challenges faced in conflict zones and humanitarian crises; and (4) Challenging deeply ingrained social stigmas through public awareness campaigns and media representation. Only through sustained advocacy, collaborative efforts, and a rights-based approach can these regions achieve genuinely equitable and inclusive societies where people with disabilities can fully participate in all aspects of life.

References

Babalola, D. O. (2012) Evaluation of global agenda: The Millennium Development Goals (MDGS).
Barbareschi, G., Carew, M. T., Johnson, E. A., Kopi, N., & Holloway, C. (2021). "When they see a wheelchair, they've not even seen me"—Factors shaping the experience of disability stigma and discrimination in Kenya. *International Journal of Environmental Research and Public Health, 18*(8), 4272. https://doi.org/10.3390/ijerph18084272
Berghs, M., Chataika, T., El-Lahib, Y., & Dube, K. (Eds.). (2020). *The Routledge handbook of disability activism*. Routledge. https://doi.org/10.4324/9781351165082
Bhattacharjee, M. (2024). Statelessness of an ethnic minority: The case of Rohingya. *Frontiers in Political Science, 6*, 1144493. https://doi.org/10.3389/fpos.2024.1144493

Bou-Karroum, L., El-Harakeh, A., Kassamany, I., Ismail, H., El Arnaout, N., Charide, R., Madi, F., Jamali, S., Martineau, T., El-Jardali, F., & Akl, E. A. (2020). Health care workers in conflict and post-conflict settings: systematic mapping of the evidence. *PloS one, 15*(5), e0233757. https://doi.org/10.1371/journal.pone.0233757

Braithwaite, J., & Mont, D. (2009). Disability and poverty: A survey of World Bank poverty assessments and implications. *Alter, 3*(3), 219–232. https://doi.org/10.1016/j.alter.2008.10.002

Cameron, C. (2016). Disability arts: the building of critical community politics and identity. In *Politics, power and community development*, 199–216. Policy Press.

Cathcart, G. S. (2016). Landmines as a form of community protection in Eastern Myanmar. *Conflict in Myanmar: War, politics, religion. ISEAS Yusof Ishak Institute, Singapore*, 121–136.

Chu, K. Y., & Gupta, S. (1998). Social safety nets in economic reform. *Social Safety Nets: Issues and Recent Experiences*.

Cook, A. D., & Ne, F. Y. (2018). Complex humanitarian emergencies and disaster management in Bangladesh: The 2017 Rohingya exodus. https://doi.org/10.13140/RG.2.2.15958.75844

Cordenillo, R., & Gardes, K. (Eds.). (2013). *Inclusive political participation and representation: The role of regional organizations*. International IDEA.

Creating an Inclusive Society: Practical Strategies to Promote Social Integration DESA. (2009).

Dahal, P., Joshi, S. K., & Swahnberg, K. (2022). A qualitative study on gender inequality and gender-based violence in Nepal. *BMC Public Health, 22*(1), 2005. https://doi.org/10.1186/s12889-022-14389-x

Das, M. B., & Espinoza, S. A. (2019). Inclusion matters in Africa. *World Bank Group*. https://doi.org/10.1596/32528

Disability, U. N. (2018). *Development report realizing the sustainable development goals by, for and with persons with disabilities*.

Dragojlović, U., Šebek, M., Mihajlović, M., Parežanin, D., Bugarčić, S., &. Petrović, D. (2009). *Pravilnici o kriterijumima za kategorizaciju sportova, misaonih sportskih igara i sportskih veština* [Regulations on the criteria for the classification of sports, thought sports games and sports skills]. MOS SSS.

Dukhan, N. (2016). *The Central African Republic crisis*. GSDRC.

Durham, J., Hill, P. S., & Hoy, D. (2013). The underreporting of landmine and explosive remnants of war injuries in Cambodia, the Lao people's democratic republic and Viet Nam. *Bulletin of the World Health Organization, 91*, 234–236. https://doi.org/10.2471/blt.12.110411

Finkelstein, V. (1980). *Attitudes and disabled people: Issues for discussion* (No. 5). World Rehabilitation Fund, Incorporated.

Gell, A. (1998). *Art and agency: An anthropological theory*. Oxford University Press.

Gerbrandt, J. S. (2009). *The experiences of people with disabilities who are on persons with disability benefits with regard to food security* (Doctoral dissertation, University of British Columbia).

Guan, Z., & Hong, F. (2016). The development of elite disability sport in China: A critical review. *The International Journal of the History of Sport, 33*(5), 485–510.

Harris, A., & Enfield, S. (2003). *Disability, equality and human rights: A training manual for development and humanitarian organisations*. Oxfam GB.

Ho, S., Eaton, S., & Mitra, M. (2020). *Civic engagement and people with disabilities: A way forward through cross-movement building*. Waltham, MA: The Lurie Institute for Disability Policy, Brandeis University. New York, NY: Ford Foundation Civic Engagement and Government Program. https://doi.org/10.48617/rpt.405

Irobi, E. (2005). Ethnic conflict management in Africa: A comparative case study of Nigeria and South Africa.

Jodell, J., & Bian, M. (2023). *Global state of inclusion in education: A review of the literature*. Special Olympics Global Center for Inclusion in Education: Washington, DC, USA.

Kabeer, N. (2005). *Social exclusion: concepts, findings and implications for the MDGs*. Paper commissioned as background for the Social Exclusion Policy Paper, Department for International Development (DFID), London.

References

Kasum, G., Strašo, G., & Nastasić-Stošković, T. (2011). Combat sports for persons with disabilities. *Physical Culture/Fizicka Kultura, 65*(1).

Katsui, H. (2005). Towards equality: Creation of the disability movement in Central Asia.

Kidd, B. (2013). Human rights and the Olympic movement after Beijing. In *Documenting the Beijing Olympics* (pp. 167–176). Routledge.

Lawson, A., & Beckett, A. E. (2021). The social and human rights models of disability: Towards a complementarity thesis. *The International Journal of Human Rights, 25*(2), 348–379. https://doi.org/10.1080/13642987.2020.1783533

Le Clair, J. (2012). *Disability in the global sport arena*. Routledge. https://doi.org/10.4324/9780203718001

Le Clair, J. M. (2009, October). Water, senses and the experiences of the pool: Paralympic athletes and swimming. In *Come to Your Senses: Creating Supportive Environments to Nurture the Sensory Capital Within. Priceedings of the 3rd International Sensory Therapy Conference*.

Le Clair, J. M. (2011). Global organizational change in sport and the shifting meaning of disability. *Sport in Society, 14*(9), 1072–1093. https://doi.org/10.1080/17430437.2011.614765

Le Roux, M. (2018). There's a place for people with disabilities within the arts: Exploring how interaction with the performing arts may facilitate the social and economic inclusion of youth with disabilities.

Louw, Q., Grimmer, K., Berner, K., Conradie, T., Bedada, D. T., & Jesus, T. S. (2021). Towards a needs-based design of the physical rehabilitation workforce in South Africa: Trend analysis [1990–2017] and a 5-year forecasting for the most impactful health conditions based on global burden of disease estimates. *BMC Public Health, 21*(1), 913. https://doi.org/10.1186/s12889-021-10962-y

Martínez-Medina, A., Morales-Calvo, S., Rodríguez-Martín, V., Meseguer-Sánchez, V., & Molina-Moreno, V. (2022). Sixteen years since the convention on the rights of persons with disabilities: What have we learned since then? *International Journal of Environmental Research and Public Health, 19*(18), 11646. https://doi.org/10.3390/ijerph191811646

Marucha, A. N., & Ngigi, S. (2018). From exclusion to inclusion: Integration of Kenya sign language during television newscasts in Kenya.

McBride-Henry, K., Nazari Orakani, S., Good, G., Roguski, M., & Officer, T. N. (2023). Disabled people's experiences accessing healthcare services during the COVID-19 pandemic: a scoping review. *BMC health services research, 23*(1), 346. https://doi.org/10.1186/s12913-023-09336-4

Mirza, M. (2011). *Unmet needs and diminished opportunities: disability, displacement and humanitarian healthcare*. UNHCR, Policy Development and Evaluation Service.

Nasrabadi, M. T., Larimian, T., Timmis, A., & Yigitcanlar, T. (2024). Mapping four decades of housing inequality research: Trends, insights, knowledge gaps, and research directions. *Sustainable Cities and Society*, 105693. https://doi.org/10.1016/j.scs.2024.105693

Rehman, M. A., Jaziri, D., & Bashir, U. (2022). Gender, disability, and social identities in tourism research in Africa: bibliometric insights. *Gender, Disability, and Tourism in Africa: Intersectional Perspectives*, 91–113. https://doi.org/10.1007/978-3-031-12551-5_5

Reilly, R. (2010). Disabilities among refugees and conflict-affected populations. *Forced Migration Review, 1*(35).

Rohwerder, B. (2013). Intellectual disabilities, violent conflict and humanitarian assistance: Advocacy of the forgotten. *Disability & Society, 28*(6), 770–783. https://doi.org/10.1080/09687599.2013.808574

Sen, A. (2000). Social exclusion: Concept, application and scrutiny. *Social Development Paper/Asian Development Bank*.

Shanmugam, M., Shivakumar, V., Anitha, V., Meenapriya, B. P., Aishwarya, S., & Anitha, R. (2014). Behavioral pattern during dental pain in intellectually disabled children: A comparative study. *International Scholarly Research Notices, 2014*(1), 824125. https://doi.org/10.1155/2014/824125

Silver, H. (2015). The contexts of social inclusion. SSRN 2641272. https://doi.org/10.2139/ssrn.2641272

Spatafora, M. N. (2021). *Education and health for inclusiveness (No. 2021/060)*. International Monetary Fund.

Spiel, C., Schwartzman, S., Busemeyer, M., Cloete, N., Drori, G., Lassnigg, L., Schober, B., Schweisfurth, M., & Verma, S. (2018). The contribution of education to social progress. https://doi.org/10.1017/9781108399661.006

Stöckl, A. (2015). Common humanity and shared destinies: Looking at the disability arts movement from an anthropological perspective. *Anthropology in Action, 21*(1), 36–43. https://doi.org/10.3167/aia.2014.210107

Tyler, J. A. (2021). *Afghanistan graveyard of empires: Why the most powerful armies of their time found only defeat or shame in this land of endless wars*. Aries Consolidated LLC.

UNICEF. (2018). *Children with disabilities in situations of armed conflict*.

United Nations. (2006). Department of Economic and social affairs disability.

Valenti, C. (2022, November). Barriers to quality education for internally displaced children. *IDMC (Internal Displacement Monitoring Centre)*.

Watermeyer, B. (Ed.). (2006). *Disability and social change: A South African agenda*. HSRC Press.

Appendices

Appendix A: Glossary of Terms

Access: The ability for individuals to obtain or use services, resources, and environments, which is significant for PwDs regarding education, healthcare, and employment.

Accommodations: Reforms or legal provisions established to empower individuals with impairments to carry out duties or participate in various activities.

Advocacy: The act of supporting a cause or proposal, particularly in promoting the rights and needs of PwDs.

Assistive Technology (AT): Tools or programs created to assist people with impairments in completing tasks that may otherwise be challenging or unfeasible.

Awareness Raising: Efforts to increase understanding and recognition of disability issues among the public.

Barrier-Free: Environments designed to eliminate physical and communal obstacles for PwDs.

Best Practices: Effective strategies and approaches have been shown to produce optimal results in disability inclusion.

Community-Based Rehabilitation (CBR): A strategy that mobilizes community resources to support and services for PwDs.

CRPD (Convention on the Rights of PwDs): An international treaty espoused by the UN to endorse and protect the rights of PwDs.

Disability Justice: A framework recognizing that PwDs are entitled to the same rights and prospects as others, focusing on equity and inclusion.

Disability Rights: The human rights of PwDs are focused on ensuring equal treatment and inclusion in all facets of life.

Disability: A bodily, cognitive, intellectual, or sensory limitation that, when combined with different obstacles, may restrict a person's complete and meaningful engagement in society.

Discrimination: Unjust or prejudicial treatment of individuals based on their disability status.

Empowerment: The process of enabling individuals to control their lives and decisions, particularly in advocating for their needs and rights.

Environmental Accessibility: The extent to which physical spaces, such as buildings and public areas, are navigable and usable for individuals with disabilities.

Equity: The fair and just treatment of all individuals, considering their specific needs and barriers, is especially relevant in policies affecting PwDs.

Inclusion: The practice of ensuring that PwDs are integrated into society and provided with equal opportunities as their non-disabled peers.

Inclusive Education: An educational approach that ensures students with disabilities take in alongside their nobles in mainstream schools with appropriate support.

Intersectionality: A framework that scrutinizes how various social identities (e.g., gender, race, disability) intersect and contribute to inimitable familiarities of oppression or indulgence.

Karma: A spiritual concept in Hinduism and Buddhism where one's actions in past lives determine present circumstances, often linked to disability perceptions in South Asia.

Legal Frameworks: The collection of laws, regulations, and guidelines that govern the rights and protections afforded to individuals with disabilities.

Medical Model of Disability: A perspective that views disability as a health condition requiring medical treatment or correction.

Mental Health: A critical aspect of wellness that encompasses emotional, psychological, and social well-being, vital for individuals with disabilities.

Mentorship: A relationship in which a more experienced individual provides guidance and support to someone with a disability.

Persons with Disabilities (PwDs): People with enduring physical, cognitive, intellectual, or sensory conditions that may limit their full and meaningful inclusion in society on an equal footing with others.

Policy: An intentional framework of guidelines designed to direct choices and attain logical results, particularly regarding disability rights and services.

Public Awareness Campaigns: Initiatives aimed at educating the public about disability issues, reducing stigma, and promoting inclusion.

Rehabilitation: Services aimed at restoring individuals with disabilities to their highest possible level of functioning and independence.

Rights-Based Approach: A framework that emphasizes recognizing and protecting the rights of PwDs and advocating for their voice and agency.

Social Model of Disability: A perception that sees disability as a result of societal barriers rather than an individual's impairment.

Social Stigma: The negative attitudes and beliefs that society holds toward individuals belonging to specific groups, including those with disabilities.

Stigma: The social discrimination and marginalization faced by individuals with disabilities due to traditional or religious beliefs.

Sustainable Development Goals (SDGs): An international structure developed by the UN that encompasses objectives aimed at promoting the inclusion and empowerment of PwDs.

Telehealth: The use of technology to provide health care from a distance is particularly beneficial for individuals with mobility challenges.

Traditional Chinese Medicine (TCM): A medical system originating in China that includes acupuncture, herbal medicine, and energy-balancing techniques, sometimes used for disability treatment.

Underrepresentation: The lack of representation of certain groups, including PwDs, in various societal sectors, such as governance and media.

Universal Design: A design strategy focused on developing products and spaces that are usable by everyone, regardless of their abilities or limitations.

Violations of Rights: Instances where the legal rights of individuals with disabilities are not upheld or respected.

Vocational Rehabilitation: Services designed to help individuals with disabilities prepare for, find, and maintain employment.

Welfare System: A government program designed to assist individuals in need, including those with disabilities, covering housing, health care, and income support.

Workplace Diversity: Including individuals from various backgrounds, including those with disabilities, in the workforce.

Appendix B: Figures and Tables

1. **Figure 1.1:** Different Types of Disabilities

   This figure categorizes disabilities into four groups: physical, mental, sensory, and intellectual disabilities. Physical disabilities affect mobility (e.g., amputation, arthritis, spinal cord injury). Mental disabilities impact cognitive function (e.g., bipolar disorder, Alzheimer's, Parkinson's disease). Sensory disabilities involve impairments like blindness, deafness, and loss of taste. Intellectual disabilities include Down syndrome, Prader-Willi syndrome, and brain injury.
2. **Figure 1.2:** Comparison of Perceptions, Beliefs, and Support Systems Surrounding Disability in Asia and Africa

   This figure compares disability perceptions in Asia and Africa, focusing on spiritual beliefs, family support, and healing practices. In Asia, disability is linked to karma, enlightenment, and filial duty, with family-based care and traditional medicine like Ayurveda and Traditional Chinese Medicine (TCM) playing key roles. In Africa, disability is often seen as an expletive or divine chastisement, leading to stigmatization but also integrated into community support. Traditional healing, including shamanic rituals and herbal medicine, is widely practiced in both regions.
3. **Figure 2.1:** Disability-Related Laws in Selected African and Asian Countries.

This figure depicts enacted laws to promote inclusion and equal rights in African nations like Uganda, Kenya, and South Africa. In Asia, countries like China, India, and Bangladesh have implemented legal frameworks such as India's Rights of PwD Act and China's Law on the Protection of Disabled Persons to enhance accessibility, education, and employment. The figure highlights regional efforts toward disability rights, inclusion, and legal protection.

4. **Figure 3.1**: Global Goals of Sustainable Development.

This figure illustrates key Sustainable Development Goals (SDGs) to foster an inclusive and equitable society. The central theme, Reduced Inequalities, emphasizes the need for accessibility and equal opportunities for all, including persons with disabilities. These elements highlight the interconnected efforts required to promote a fair, sustainable, and inclusive world. The visual representation reinforces the importance of global collaboration in achieving these objectives.

5. **Figure 4.1**: Various Tools and Software Used to Enhance Accessibility for People with Disabilities.

The figure illustrates the technological advancements in assistive technology for people with disabilities across Asia and Africa. The left side represents Asian innovations, including AI-powered wheelchairs, prosthetic hands, brain-computer interfaces, AI hearing aids, and prosthetic lenses. The right side highlights African assistive technologies, such as the ShazaCin App, the IXAM platform for visual impairments, AI-powered magnifiers, smart bracelets, and advanced prosthetic limbs. The central AI symbol signifies the role of artificial intelligence in enhancing accessibility and independence for individuals with disabilities in both regions.

6. **Figure 5.1**: Concept of Social Inclusion for Individuals with Disabilities.

The figure highlights community participation, emphasizing integrating PwDs into the populace. Accessible transportation is depicted as a crucial factor in ensuring mobility through adapted vehicles. The role of AI in assistive technology is also showcased, demonstrating how AI-powered innovations enhance accessibility and independence. Additionally, the image includes wheelchair accessibility, underscoring the importance of inclusive infrastructure. It also acknowledges neurological and motor disabilities, representing the challenges faced by individuals with movement disorders. Furthermore, elderly and mobility support are depicted through assistive devices like walkers, catering to seniors and individuals with limited mobility.

7. **Table 1.1**: Cultural Perspectives, Modern Beliefs, Societal Views, and Actions Taken Regarding Disability in Asia and Africa
8. **Table 3.1**: Key Challenges and Aspects of Inclusive Education for PwDs Across Different Regions
9. **Table 4.1**: Various Software Developments Designed to Enhance Accessibility for People with Disabilities in Public Spaces

10. **Table 5.1**: Global Disability Rights Issues, Focusing on Civic Engagement, Intersectionality, and Policy Advocacy

Appendix C: Methodological and Cultural Considerations

1. The chapters relied on a qualitative literature review from various disciplines, including sociology, psychology, and public health, offering a comprehensive perspective on disability rights and technology's role within this context.
2. Acknowledging the diverse cultural interpretations of disability within different communities is paramount for effectively implementing inclusive practices. Understanding local beliefs and values can enhance engagement and support for PwDs.

Appendix D: Relevant Frameworks and Policies

1. The Convention on the Rights of PwDs (CRPD) serves as an all-inclusive international framework to endorse and screen the rights of PwDs.
2. Regional Policies: Various Asian and African nations have developed frameworks underpinned by international guidelines, focusing on inclusive education, accessible infrastructure, and economic empowerment for PwDs.

Appendix E: Statistical Insights

1. The prevalence of disability in developing regions is reported to affect over 15% of the population, with significant variations based on socioeconomic factors and access to healthcare.
2. In many countries, over 90% of children with disabilities do not attend school, highlighting a critical area for intervention through inclusive education policies.

The manufacturer's authorised representative in the EU is Springer Nature Customer Service Centre GmbH, Europaplatz 3, 69115 Heidelberg, Germany. If you have any concerns regarding our products, please contact ProductSafety@springernature.com

Printed and bound by CPI Group (UK) Ltd, Croydon, CR0 4YY

26/03/2026

02078953-0015